Type 1 Diabetes Cookbook For Seniors

Easy Meals To Manage Blood Sugar

And Boost Well-Being

Dr. Josephine S. Sanger

Table of Contents

Introduction

"The Type 1 Diabetes Cookbook for Seniors" – a guide meant to empower and

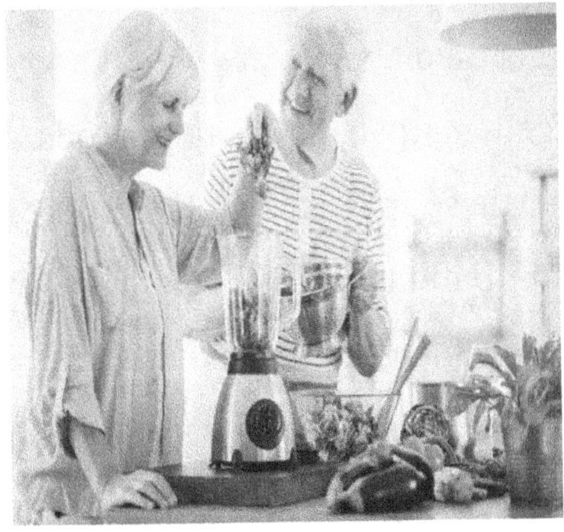

inspire seniors on their journey to managing diabetes through the transformative power of diet. In this unique culinary exploration, we dig into the art of producing delectable and healthy meals specifically designed to satisfy thc nccds of persons navigating Type 1 Diabetes in their golden years.

As we age, the necessity of a well-balanced diet becomes vital, and for people with Type

1 Diabetes, it becomes a crucial component in sustaining a healthy and vibrant lifestyle. This cookbook is a compilation of recipes; it's a comprehensive resource that blends the newest insights on diabetes care with the joy of tasting excellent, diabetic-friendly foods.

Throughout these pages, you'll discover smart tips on building a diabetes-friendly kitchen, understanding the complexities of a senior-specific diet, and creating meals that not only support blood sugar stability but also bring joy to the dining table. Whether you're newly diagnosed or have been managing diabetes for years, this cookbook acts as your trusty companion, delivering a rich tapestry of recipes, meal plans, and practical guidance to make every mouthful a step toward a better, more fulfilled life. Let's go on this culinary journey together, embracing the nourishing power of food in the pursuit of a healthy and flourishing life with Type 1 Diabetes.

Why Nutrition Matters in Type 1 Diabetes

Nutrition is a vital factor that plays a pivotal part in the overall treatment and well-being of individuals with this condition. Here are numerous fundamental reasons why nutrition is of vital importance:

- Blood Sugar Control: Proper eating is crucial in regulating blood sugar levels. The type and quantity of food ingested immediately impact glucose levels, making balanced meals vital for averting spikes and crashes.

- Energy and Nutrient Needs: Seniors, in particular, have specific nutritional requirements. A well-balanced diet ensures the elderly to acquire the required nutrients for energy, immunological support, and overall health, helping battle any issues connected with diabetes.

- Weight Management: Maintaining a healthy weight is essential in managing Type 1 Diabetes. Nutrition regulates weight, and a balanced diet can aid in weight control, minimizing the risk of complications connected to obesity or underweight concerns.

- Cardiovascular Health: Diabetes raises the risk of cardiovascular issues. A heart-healthy diet, low in saturated fats and sodium, can decrease these risks and contribute to overall cardiovascular well-being.

- Preventing Complications: Proper diet improves overall health and helps prevent diabetes-related complications, such as kidney disease, nerve damage, and visual issues. A nutrient-rich diet is a proactive approach to long-term well-being.

- Glycemic Index Awareness: Understanding the glycemic index of foods is vital. Nutrition choices that favor low-glycemic meals can help maintain stable blood sugar levels, enabling improved diabetes management.

- Digestive Health: Diabetes might impact digestion. A diet high in fiber and readily digestible foods supports gastrointestinal health, contributing to the prevention of digestive disorders typically associated with diabetes.

- Enhancing Quality of Life: Optimal nutrition contributes to an improved quality of life. It offers the required fuel for daily tasks, raises energy levels, and positively influences mental well-being.

Chapter 1:Basics of Type 1 Diabetes

Type 1 Diabetes is a chronic autoimmune illness characterized by the immune system's attack on the insulin-producing beta cells in

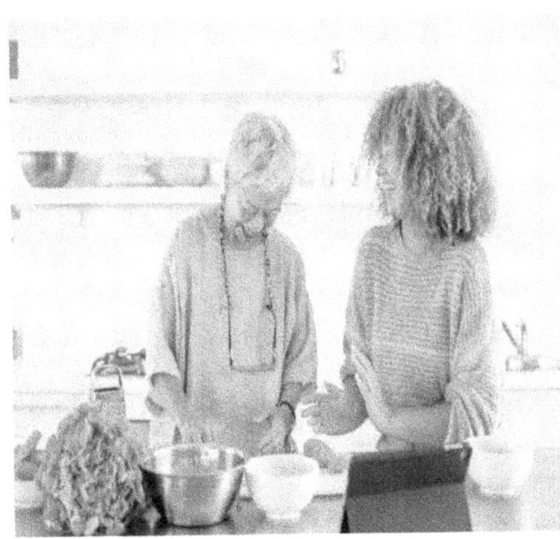

the pancreas. This leads to little or no insulin synthesis, a hormone crucial for regulating blood sugar (glucose) levels.

Symptoms: Common symptoms of Type 1 Diabetes include increased thirst (polydipsia), frequent urination (polyuria), unexplained weight loss, excessive appetite (polyphagia), and exhaustion. Prompt detection of these symptoms is critical for early diagnosis and action.

Blood Sugar Monitoring and Management:

Regular monitoring is vital to check blood sugar levels and make informed decisions regarding insulin dosage, nutrition, and lifestyle.

- *Glucose Meters:* Portable devices allow individuals to measure their blood sugar levels with a small blood sample.

Factors Contributing to Diabetes:

1. ***Genetic Predisposition:*** A family history of diabetes can raise the risk.
- ***Preventive Measures:*** Regular health check-ups and awareness of family history. Implementing a healthy

lifestyle is crucial even with a genetic tendency.

2. ***Lifestyle Choices:*** Sedentary lifestyle, poor dietary habits, and excessive consumption of processed foods lead to the development of diabetes.

- ***Preventive Measures:*** Engage in regular physical activity, adopt a balanced and nutritious diet, restrict processed and sugary foods, and maintain a healthy weight.

3. ***Obesity:*** Excess body weight, especially in the abdomen area, is a substantial risk factor for diabetes.

- Preventive Measures: Achieve and maintain a healthy weight through a mix of regular exercise and a well-balanced diet.

4. *Age and Ethnicity:* The risk of diabetes increases with age, and certain ethnic groups are more susceptible.

- ***Preventive Measures:*** While age and ethnicity cannot be changed, a healthy lifestyle can attenuate the impact and reduce the total risk.

5. *Hormonal Changes:* Certain hormonal conditions or alterations, such as polycystic ovarian syndrome (PCOS), might contribute to insulin resistance.

- ***Preventive Measures:*** Managing hormonal problems through medical guidance and establishing a healthy lifestyle.

Strategies to Avoid Diabetes:

> Healthy Diet: Emphasize whole foods, fruits, vegetables, whole grains, lean meats, and healthy fats.

Action: Limit intake of processed meals, sugary beverages, and refined carbs.

> Regular Physical Activity: Aim for at least 150 minutes of moderate-intensity exercise per week.

Action: Incorporate a variety of physical activities, including aerobic exercises and strength training.

> ***Regular Health Check-ups:*** Schedule routine check-ups to monitor blood sugar levels, especially if there is a family history or other risk factors.

Action: Stay informed about health status and follow medical advice.

➢ *Limit Alcohol Consumption:* Moderation in alcohol consumption is advised.

Action: Be careful of alcohol intake and its potential impact on blood sugar levels.

➢ *Stress Management:* Adopt stress-reducing hobbies such as meditation, yoga, or mindfulness.

Action: Prioritize mental well-being and identify effective ways to manage stress.

Chapter 2: Nutrients Essential for Seniors with Type 1 Diabetes

Nutrient needs for seniors with diabetes

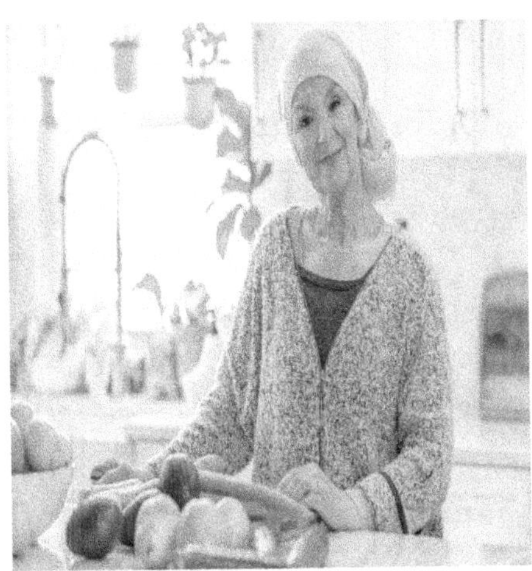

play a critical role in maintaining overall health and regulating blood sugar levels. Here are major nutrients, their importance, and food sources acceptable for seniors with diabetes:

Fiber:

- *Importance:* Aids in digestion, helps control blood sugar levels, and improves heart health.

- *Food Sources:* Whole grains (brown rice, quinoa, oats)
- Legumes (beans, lentils)
- Vegetables (broccoli, Brussels sprouts)
- Fruits (apples, berries, pears)

Protein:

- *Importance:* Essential for muscle upkeep, immunological function, and blood sugar management.
- *Food Sources:* Lean meats (chicken, turkey, fish)
- Legumes and beans
- Low-fat dairy products (Greek yogurt, cottage cheese)

Tofu and other plant-based protein sources

Healthy Fats:

- *Importance:* Supports heart health and gives sustained energy.
- *Food Sources:* Avocado Nuts and seeds (almonds, walnuts, chia seeds)
- ***Olive oil:*** Fatty fish (salmon, mackerel)

<u>Vitamins and Minerals:</u>

- *Importance:* Essential for different body functions, including immune support and bone health.
- *Food Sources:* Colorful vegetables (leafy greens, carrots, bell peppers)
- Fruits (citrus fruits, berries)

Dairy or fortified plant-based milk for vitamin D and calcium

Nuts and seeds for magnesium and zinc

<u>Antioxidants:</u>

- *Importance:* Help battle oxidative stress and inflammation.
- *Food Sources:* Berries (blueberries, strawberries)
- Dark leafy greens (kale, spinach)
- Dark chocolate (in moderation)
- Green tea

Omega-3 Fatty Acids:

- *Importance:* Support heart health and provide anti-inflammatory properties.
- *Food Sources:* Fatty fish (salmon, trout)
- Chia seeds and flaxseeds
- Walnuts

Calcium:

- *Importance:* Essential for bone health.

- *Food Sources:* Low-fat or fat-free dairy products (milk, yogurt)
- Leafy greens (kale, broccoli)

Fortified plant-based milk (almond, soy)

Magnesium:

- *Importance:* Supports muscle and nerve function, and blood glucose regulation.
- *Food Sources:* Nuts and seeds (almonds, pumpkin seeds)
- Leafy greens (spinach, Swiss chard) Whole grains

Hydration:

- *Importance:* Helps maintain healthy bodily processes and maintains kidney health.
- Hydration Sources: Water, Herbal teas

- Low-sugar electrolyte-rich beverages

<u>Potassium:</u>

- *Importance:* Supports heart health and helps regulate blood pressure.
- *Food Sources:* Bananas
- Oranges Potatoes (with skin)

Diabetes Kitchen Essentials:

★ Measuring Cups and Spoons: Precise portion management is vital for managing carbohydrate consumption. Measuring instruments assist ensure consistency in portion amounts.

★ Food Scale: Weighing food can provide accurate carbohydrate counts, resulting in better insulin dosage estimates and blood sugar management.

★ Quality Cookware: Invest in non-stick pans, excellent pots, and bakeware for healthier cooking with minimum need for extra fats.

★ Blender or Food Processor: Ideal for producing healthful smoothies, soups, and sauces utilizing whole, unprocessed foods.

★ Slow Cooker or Instant Pot: Convenient for creating healthy meals with lean proteins, whole grains, and plenty of vegetables.

★ Vegetable Spiralizer: Creates vegetable noodles as a low-carb alternative to typical pasta, promoting a balanced diet.

★ Herbs and Spices: Enhance flavor without adding excessive salt or sugar, making meals appealing for persons with diabetes.

★ Olive Oil with Vinegar: A heart-healthy alternative to saturated fats for cooking and salad dressings.

★ Nut and Seed Butter: Provides healthy fats and proteins, perfect for spreads, snacks, and smoothies.

★ Low-Sodium Broths: Adds flavor to foods without excess salt, a crucial aspect for regulating blood pressure.

★ Sugar Substitutes: Allows for sweetness in recipes without increasing blood sugar levels; examples include stevia or erythritol.

★ Whole Grain Flours: Substituting refined flours with whole grain choices aids in better blood sugar regulation.

Diabetes-Friendly Ingredients:

1. Lean Proteins: Chicken breast, turkey, salmon, tofu, and beans.

- Supports muscle health and delivers sustained energy without excessive saturated fats.

2. Non-Starchy Vegetables: Leafy greens, broccoli, cauliflower, bell peppers.

- Low in carbohydrates, high in fiber, and rich in important nutrients.

3. Healthy Fats: Avocado, olive oil, almonds, seeds, fatty seafood.

- Provides necessary fatty acids and improves heart health.

4. Whole Fruits: Berries, apples, and citrus fruits.

- Provides natural sweetness along with fiber and important vitamins.

5. Whole Grains: Quinoa, brown rice, whole wheat.

6. High in fiber and minerals, encouraging stable blood sugar levels.

7. Eggs: A flexible protein source ideal for numerous meals.

8. Herbs and Spices: Cinnamon, turmeric, basil, garlic. Adds flavor without added calories, sugar, or sodium.

9. Sugar-Free Condiments: Mustard, hot sauce, salsa. Enhances taste without extra sugars or bad fats.

Chapter 3: Meal planning

Creating a well-balanced diet plan is vital for those with Type 1 Diabetes to maintain

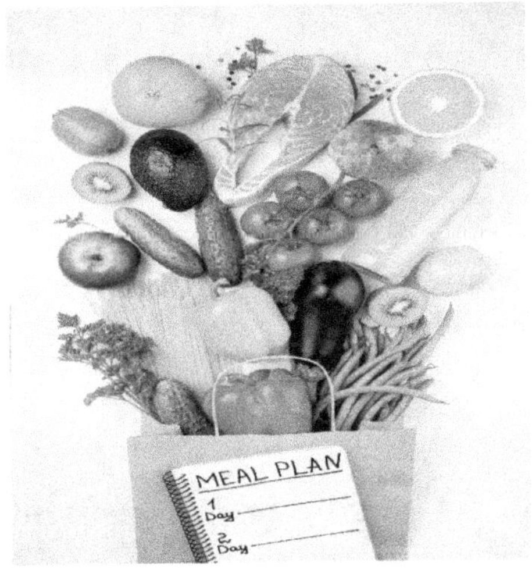

blood sugar levels efficiently. Here's a guide on type 1 diabetic meal planning:

→ Consistent Carbohydrate Intake: Consistency in carbohydrate intake assists in improved insulin regulation. Spread carbohydrates evenly among meals and snacks.

→ Balanced Meals: Include a balance of carbohydrates, proteins, and healthy fats in each meal. This combination assists in balancing blood sugar levels and gives continuous energy.

→ Portion Control: Be aware of portion sizes to avoid overconsumption of carbs, which can contribute to rises in blood sugar levels.

→ Timing Matters: Space out meals and snacks appropriately throughout the day to minimize big spikes or decreases in blood sugar. Consistent meal time promotes insulin regulation.

→ Smart Snacking: Choose snacks that mix protein and fiber to give sustained energy and reduce blood sugar changes between meals.

→ Mindful Eating: Practice mindful eating by paying attention to hunger and fullness signs. Avoid distractions during meals to build a deeper connection with food.

→ Plan: Plan meals and snacks to ensure access to diabetes-friendly options and avoid impulsive food decisions.

14-Day Meal Plan

Day 1:

Breakfast:

- Scrambled eggs with spinach and tomatoes
- Greek yogurt with a handful of berries

Lunch:

- Grilled chicken salad with mixed greens, cucumbers, and vinaigrette dressing (Quinoa or brown rice on the side)

Dinner:

- Baked salmon with lemon and herbs
- Steamed broccoli and cauliflower
- Sweet potato wedges

Snack:

- Celery sticks with hummus

Day 2:

Breakfast:

- Oatmeal topped with chopped almonds and fresh fruit
- Low-fat milk or enriched plant-based milk

Lunch:

- Turkey and avocado whole-grain wrap

- Mixed green salad with balsamic vinaigrette

Dinner:

- Stir-fried tofu with colorful veggies (bell peppers, snap peas, carrots)
- Serve with Quinoa or cauliflower rice

Snack:

- Handful of walnuts

Day 3:

Breakfast:

- Whole-grain waffles with sugar-free syrup
- Cottage cheese with sliced peaches

Lunch:

- Lentil soup Whole-grain roll on the side

Dinner:

- Grilled shrimp skewers
- Quinoa pilaf

Snack:

- Apple slices with almond butter

<u>Day 4:</u>

Breakfast:

- Smoothie with spinach, banana, Greek yogurt, and chia seeds
- Hard-boiled egg

Lunch:

- Quinoa salad (Grilled chicken breast on top)

Dinner:

- Baked cod with lemon and dill
- Roasted Brussels sprouts
- Wild rice

Snack:

- Sugar-free yogurt with a sprinkling of cinnamon

<u>*Day 5:*</u>

Breakfast:

- Vegetable and cheese omelet
- Whole-grain bread with avocado

Lunch:

- Chickpea salad (Whole-grain pita on the side)

Dinner:

- Beef stir-fry with broccoli, bell peppers, and snap peas served with Cauliflower rice

Snack:

- Sliced cucumber with tzatziki

<u>Day 6:</u>

Breakfast:

- Whole-grain pancakes with sugar-free syrup (Mixed berries on top)

Lunch:

- Spinach and feta-filled chicken breast
- Quinoa salad with cranberries and almonds

Dinner:

- Grilled vegetable skewers (zucchini, mushrooms, cherry tomatoes)
- Baked chicken thighs with rosemary

Snack:

- Sugar-free gelatin with whipped cream

<u>Day 7:</u>

Breakfast:

- Cottage cheese with pineapple parfait

- Whole-grain English muffin with cream cheese

Lunch:

- Turkey and veggie kebabs

- Quinoa tabbouleh

Dinner:

- Baked tilapia with garlic and herbs

- Steamed green beans

- Sweet potato mash

Snack:

- Handful of mixed nuts

Day 8:

Breakfast:

- Greek yogurt parfait with sliced strawberries and a sprinkle of granola

- Whole-grain English muffin with peanut butter

Lunch:

- Lentil and vegetable soup
- Quinoa salad with sliced cucumber, cherry tomatoes, and feta

Dinner:

- Grilled chicken breast with a lemon-herb marinade
- Roasted sweet potatoes

Snack:

- Sugar-free fruit popsicle

Day 9:

Breakfast:

- Scrambled eggs with sautéed spinach and whole-grain bread
- Fresh orange slices

Lunch:

- Turkey and avocado lettuce wrap
- Quinoa and black bean salad

Dinner:

- Baked cod with tomato and olive relish
- Cauliflower mash

Snack:

- Carrot sticks with hummus

Day 10:

Breakfast:

- Smoothie with kale, banana, and a scoop of protein powder
- Whole-grain bagel with cream cheese

Lunch:

- Chickpea and vegetable stir-fry with tofu

- Brown rice on the side

Dinner:

- Grilled fish with a honey-mustard glaze
- Roasted Brussels sprouts
- Quinoa pilaf

Snack:

- Cottage cheese with sliced peaches

Day 11:

Breakfast:

- Whole-grain French toast with sliced strawberries
- Hard-boiled egg

Lunch:

- Caprese salad with tomatoes, fresh mozzarella, and basil
- Whole-grain crackers on the side

Dinner:

- Beef and veggie kebabs with a soy-ginger marinade
- Cauliflower rice

Snack:

- Handful of mixed berries

Day 12:

Breakfast:

- Overnight oats
- Scrambled eggs with chopped tomatoes

Lunch:

- Quinoa and black bean stuffed peppers
- Greek salad with olives and feta

Dinner:

- Baked chicken thighs with rosemary and garlic and Steamed green beans
- Quinoa pilaf

Snack:

- Sugar-free yogurt with a sprinkling of cinnamon

Day 13:

Breakfast:

- Whole-grain waffles with sugar-free syrup
- Sliced kiwi on the side

Lunch:

- Turkey and vegetable stir-fry with broccoli and bell peppers
- Brown rice

Dinner:

- Grilled veggie and chicken skewers

- Quinoa tabbouleh

Snack:

- Celery sticks with almond butter

<u>*Day 14:*</u>

Breakfast:

- Vegetable and cheese frittata
- Whole-grain toast with avocado

Lunch:

- Spinach and strawberry salad with grilled chicken
- Whole-grain roll on the side

Dinner:

- Baked tilapia with lemon and dill
- Roasted sweet potato wedges

Snack:

- Sugar-free gelatin with whipped cream

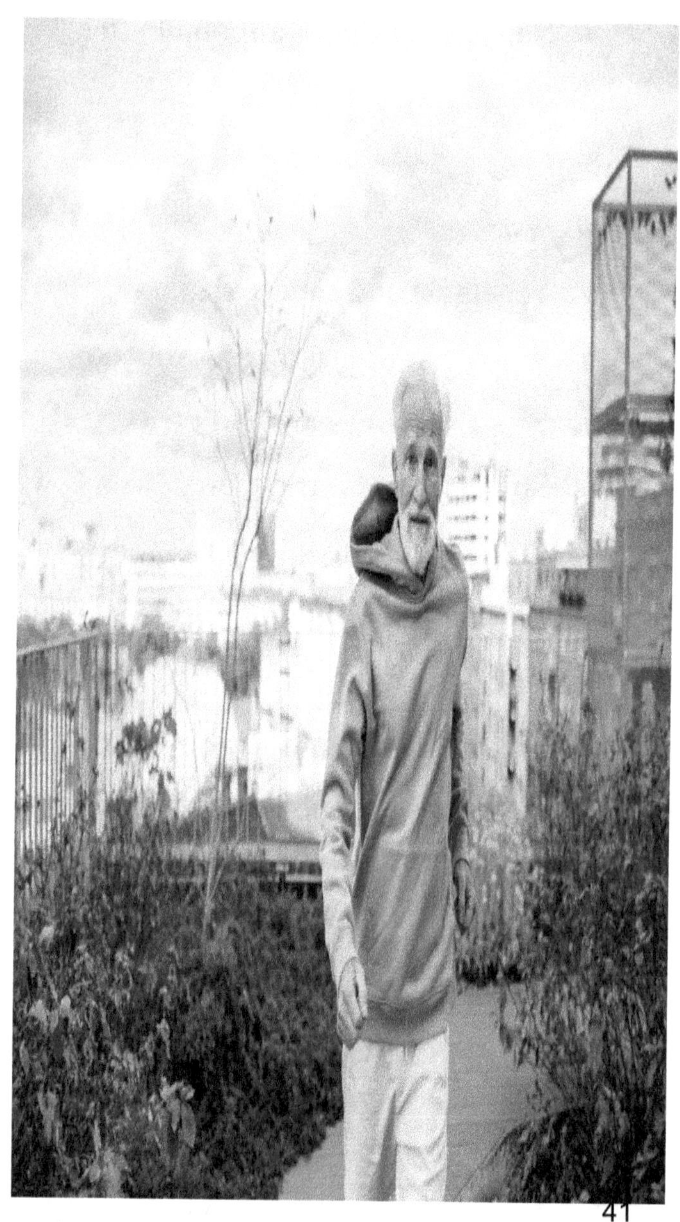

Chapter 4: Diabetes Diets Recipes

Breakfast Recipes:

Scrambled Eggs with Spinach and Tomatoes

Ingredients:

2 big eggs

1 cup fresh spinach, chopped

1/2 cup cherry tomatoes, halved

1 tablespoon olive oil

Salt and pepper to taste

Preparation:

1. Warm your olive oil in a non-stick skillet over medium heat.

2. Put cherry tomatoes and sauté until slightly softened.

3. Add chopped spinach to the skillet and simmer until wilted.

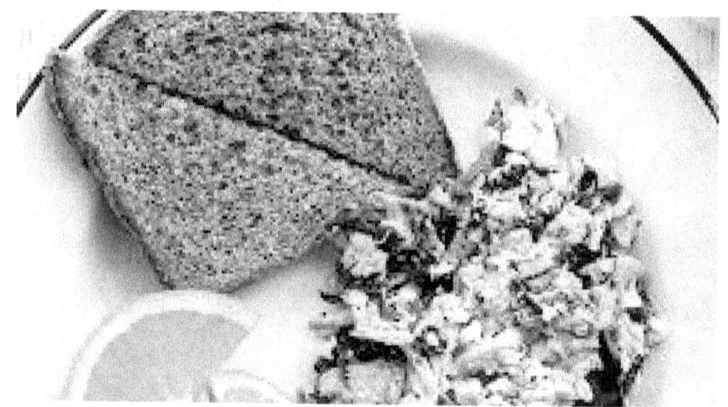

4. In a bowl, whisk the eggs and add a little salt and pepper.

5. Pour the eggs over the vegetables in the skillet.

6. Mix the eggs and vegetables until the eggs are cooked through.

7. Eat hot, and optionally garnish with fresh herbs.

Whole-grain waffles with Sugar-Free Syrup

Ingredients:

1 cup whole-grain waffle mix

1 cup water or milk (according to waffle mix
specifications)

Cooking spray

Sugar-free syrup

Preparation:

1. Warm your waffle iron according to
   the manufacturer's directions.

2. In a bowl, mix the whole-grain waffle
   mix with water or milk until
   completely blended.

3. Lightly coat the waffle iron with
   cooking spray.

4. Pour the waffle batter onto the
   preheated iron and cook according to
   the manufacturer's directions until
   golden brown.

5. Serve the whole-grain waffles with sugar-free syrup.

Cottage Cheese and Pineapple Parfait

Ingredients:

1/2 cup low-fat cottage cheese

1/2 cup fresh pineapple chunks

1/4 cup granola (select a low-sugar alternative)

1 tablespoon shredded coconut (unsweetened)

1 teaspoon honey (optional)

Preparation:

1. In a serving glass or bowl, layer half of the low-fat cottage cheese.

2. Add half of the fresh pineapple chunks.

3. Sprinkle half of the granola and shredded coconut.

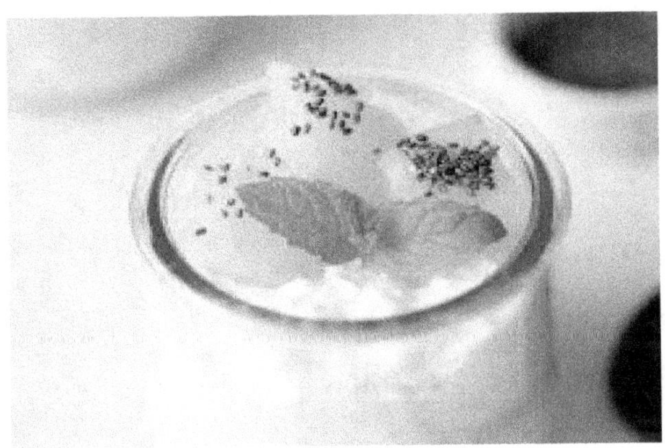

4. Repeat the layering with the remaining ingredients.
5. Drizzle with honey if preferred.
6. Serve immediately and enjoy this refreshing parfait.

Serving: 1 serving

Nutritional Value (Approximate):

- Calories: 250
- Carbohydrates: 30g

- Protein: 15g

- Healthy Fats: ~8g

- Fiber: ~4g

<u>Vegetable and Cheese Frittata</u>

Ingredients:

4 big eggs

1/2 cup bell peppers, diced

1/2 cup cherry tomatoes, halved

1/4 cup red onions, diced

Shredded Cheese

1/4 cup (cheddar or your choice)

1 tablespoon olive oil

Salt and pepper to taste

Fresh herbs for garnish (optional)

Preparation:

1. Set the oven to 350°F (180°C).

2. In a bowl, whisk the eggs and add a little salt and pepper.

3. Warm your olive oil in an oven-safe skillet over medium heat.

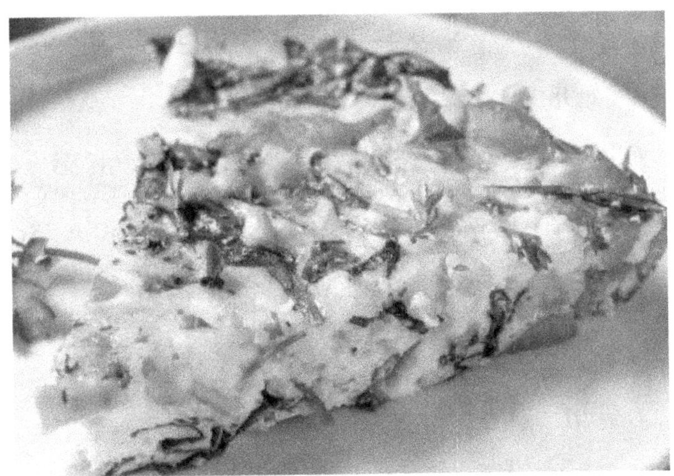

4. Pour in chopped bell peppers, cherry tomatoes, and red onions into the skillet. Sauté until vegetables are slightly softened.

5. Add the whisked eggs over the vegetables in the skillet.

6. Let the eggs set around the edges.

7. Add drops of shredded cheese evenly over the frittata.

8. Transfer the skillet to the preheated oven and bake for 10-12 minutes or until the frittata is set and the cheese is melted.

9. Decorate with fresh herbs if desired.

10. Slice and serve the veggie and cheese frittata.

Cooking Time: Prep Time: 10 minutes
Cooking Time: 12 minutes in the oven
Serving: 2 servings
Nutritional Value (Approximate):

- Calories: 300

- Carbohydrates: 10g, Protein: 20g

- Healthy Fats: 20g, Fiber: 3g

Veggie Omelet with Whole-Grain Toast

Ingredients:

2 big eggs

1/4 cup chopped bell peppers (mixed colors)

1/4 cup chopped tomatoes

1/4 cup chopped spinach

1 tablespoon diced onions

1 teaspoon olive oil

Salt and pepper to taste

Preparation:

1. Warm your olive oil in a non-stick skillet over medium heat.

2. Sauté onions until transparent, then add bell peppers, tomatoes, and spinach. Allow to cook for 2-3 minutes until vegetables are soft.

3. In a bowl, whisk eggs and add salt and pepper.

4. Pour in the eggs over the vegetables in the skillet, turning to thoroughly distribute.

5. Allow to cook until the edges firm, then gently lift the edges to enable raw eggs to flow below.

6. Once the omelet is ready, fold it in half and place it onto a plate.

7. Serve with a slice of whole-grain bread.

Preparation Time:4 minutes

Serving: 1

Nutritional Value:

- Calories: 250

- Carbohydrates: 10g, Protein: 15g

- Healthy Fats: 15g, Fiber: 2g

Greek Yogurt Parfait with Berries and Almonds

Ingredients:

1/2 cup Greek yogurt (unsweetened)

1/4 cup blueberries

1/4 cup strawberries, sliced

1 tablespoon almonds, chopped

1 teaspoon honey (optional)

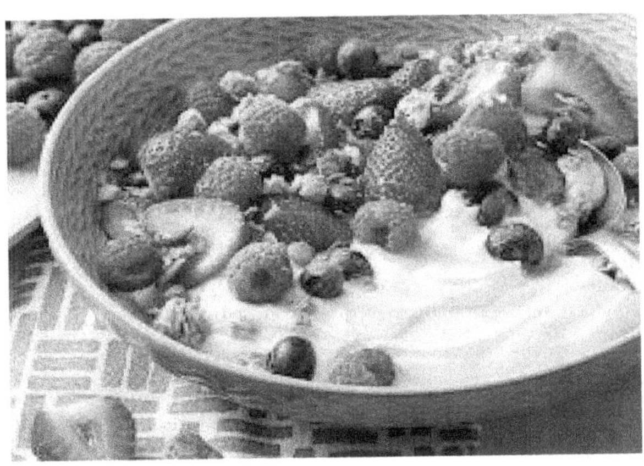

Preparation:

1. In a serving glass or bowl, layer half of the Greek yogurt.

2. Add half of the blueberries and strawberries.

3. Repeat with the remaining yogurt and berries.

4. Sprinkle chopped almonds on top.

5. Pour a little honey if preferred. Before serving.

Serving: 1

Nutritional Value:

- Calories: 200, Carbohydrates: 20g
- Protein: ~15g, Healthy Fats: ~8g
- Fiber: 3g

Whole-grain pancakes with Sliced Peaches

Ingredients:

1/2 cup whole-grain pancake mix

1/3 cup low-fat milk or almond milk

1/2 teaspoon vanilla extract

1 teaspoon canola oil

1 small peach, cut

Preparation:

1. In a bowl, mix pancake mix, milk, and vanilla extract until completely blended.

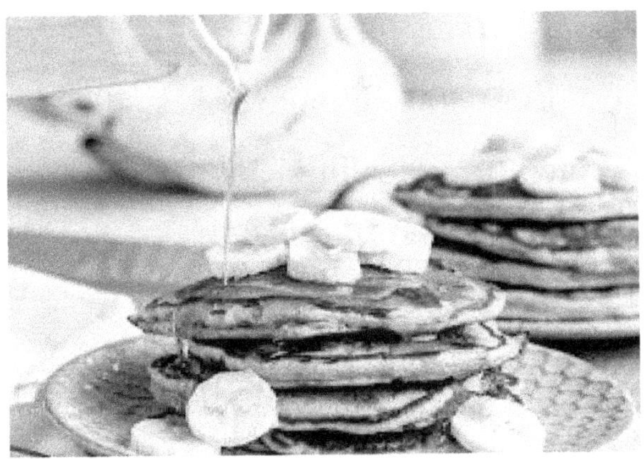

2. Heat a griddle or non-stick pan over medium heat and add canola oil.

3. Pour in a 1/4 cup of batter onto the griddle for each pancake.

4. Allow to cook until bubbles appear on the surface, then turn and cook the other side until golden brown.

5. Serve with sliced peaches on top.

Cooking Time: 15 minutes

Serving: 2

Nutritional Value:

- Calories: 300, Carbohydrates: 40g
- Protein: 8g, Healthy Fats: 10g
- Fiber: 6g

Overnight Chia Seed Pudding with Mixed Berries

Ingredients:

2 tablespoons chia seeds

1/2 cup unsweetened almond milk

1/2 teaspoon vanilla extract

1/4 cup raspberries

1/4 cup blackberries

1 tablespoon unsweetened shredded coconut

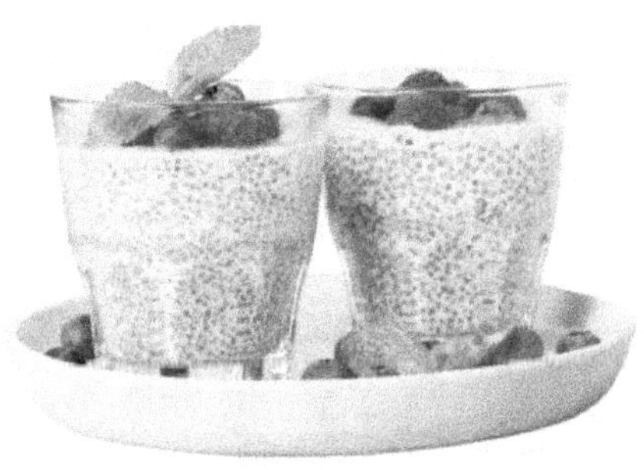

Preparation:

1. In a bowl, mix chia seeds, almond milk, and vanilla essence.

2. Mix well and allow it to refrigerate overnight or for at least 4 hours.

3. Before serving, layer with raspberries, blackberries, and shredded coconut.

Serving: 1

Nutritional Value:

- Calories: 180

- Carbohydrates: 20g, Protein: 5g
- Healthy Fats: 10g, Fiber: 10g

Spinach and Feta Breakfast Wrap

Ingredients:

1 whole-grain tortilla

2 big eggs, scrambled

1 cup fresh spinach leaves

2 tablespoons feta cheese, crumbled

1 teaspoon olive oil

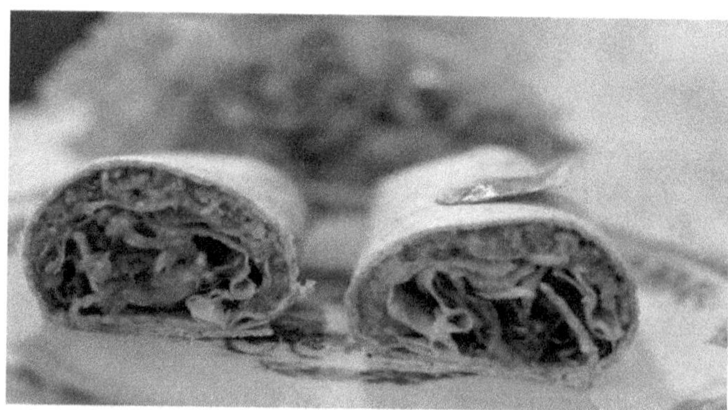

Preparation:

1. In a pan, heat olive oil over medium heat.

2. Add fresh spinach leaves and sauté until wilted.

3. Remove spinach from the skillet and put aside.

4. In the same pan, scramble the eggs.

5. Warm the tortilla and construct by layering scrambled eggs, sautéed spinach, and crumbled feta in the center.

6. Fold into a wrap and serve.

Cooking Time: 5 minutes

Serving: 1

Nutritional Value:

- Calories: 280
- Carbohydrates: 20g
- Protein: 15g, Healthy Fats: 15g, Fiber: 4g

Almond Butter and Banana Smoothie

Ingredients:

1 cup unsweetened almond milk

1 medium banana

1 tbsp almond butter

1/2 teaspoon cinnamon

Ice cubes (optional)

Preparation:

1. In a blender, combine almond milk, banana, almond butter, and cinnamon.
2. Blend until smooth.
3. Add ice cubes if required and mix again.
4. Pour into a glass and enjoy.

Serving: 1

Nutritional Value:

- Calories: 250
- Carbohydrates: 30g, Protein: 7g
- Healthy Fats: 12g, Fiber: 5g

Berry and Almond Oatmeal Bowl

Ingredients:

1/2 cup rolled oats

1 cup unsweetened almond milk

1/4 cup mixed berries (strawberries, blueberries, raspberries)

1 tablespoon almonds, sliced

1/2 teaspoon cinnamon

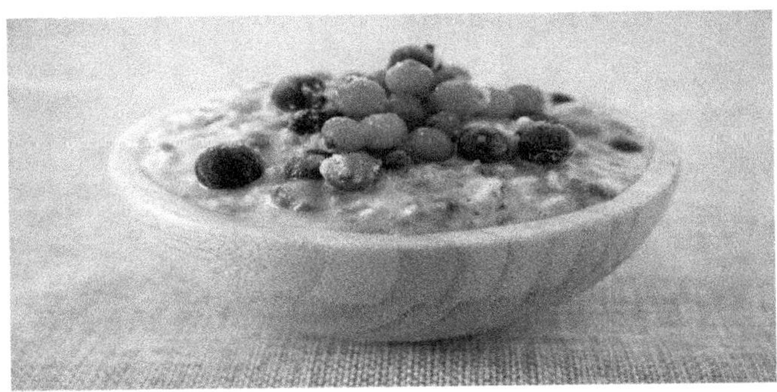

Preparation:

1. In a saucepan, combine rolled oats and almond milk.

2. Allow to cook over medium heat until the oats are cooked and the mixture thickens.

3. Transfer the oats to a bowl and top with mixed berries, sliced almonds, and a sprinkling of cinnamon.

Cooking Time: 5 minutes

Serving: 1

Nutritional Value:

- Calories: 280 Carbohydrates: 40g
- Protein: 8g, Healthy Fats: 10g
- Fiber: 8g

Avocado and Tomato Breakfast Toast

Ingredients:

1 slice of whole-grain bread

1/2 avocado, mashed

1 small tomato, sliced

1 teaspoon olive oil

Salt and pepper to taste

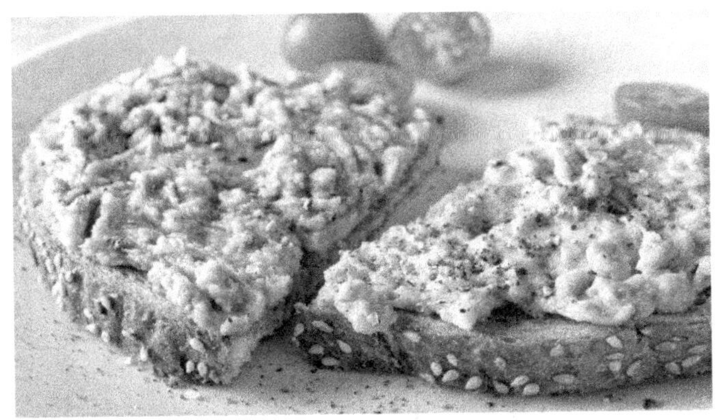

Preparation:

1. Toast the whole-grain bread slice.

2. Spread mashed avocado over the bread.

3. Top with sliced tomatoes.

4. Add a drop of olive oil and season with salt and pepper.

Serving: 1

Nutritional Value:

Calories: ~220 Carbohydrates: ~20g

Protein: ~5g

Healthy Fats: ~15g

Fiber: ~6g

Cinnamon Apple Cottage Cheese Bowl

Ingredients:

1/2 cup low-fat cottage cheese

1 medium apple, diced

1 tablespoon chopped walnuts

1/2 teaspoon cinnamon

1 teaspoon honey (optional)

Preparation:

1. In a bowl, combine cottage cheese, diced apple, and chopped walnuts.

2. Sprinkle with cinnamon and combine well.

3. Drizzle with honey if preferred.

Serving: 1

Nutritional Value:

- Calories: 230
- Carbohydrates: 25g, Protein: 10g
- Healthy Fats: 10g, Fiber: 4g

Lunch Recipes:

Spinach and Strawberry Salad with Grilled Chicken

Ingredients:

4 ounces boneless, skinless chicken breast

3 cups fresh spinach leaves

1 cup strawberries, cut

1/4 cup red onion, finely sliced

1/4 cup feta cheese, crumbled

2 tablespoons balsamic vinaigrette dressing (low-sugar)

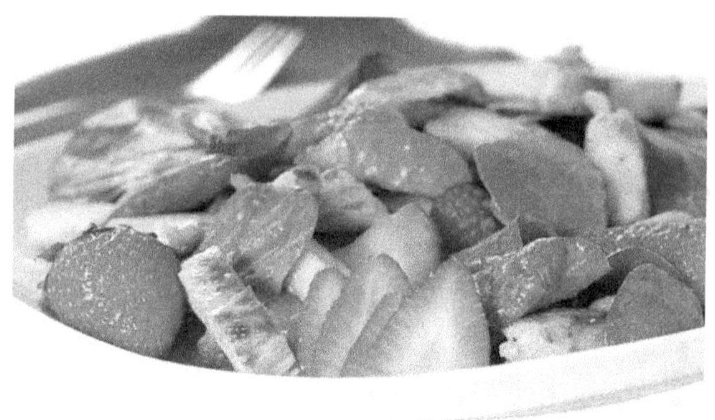

Preparation:

1. Apply salt and pepper to the chicken.

2. Grill the chicken until fully done.

3. In a large bowl, add fresh spinach, sliced strawberries, red onion, and feta cheese.

4. Slice grilled chicken and place on top of the salad.

5. Drizzle with balsamic vinaigrette dressing before serving.

Cooking Time: Prep Time: 10 minutes

Grill Time: 15 minutes

Serving: 1

Nutritional Value (Approximate):

- Calories: 350
- Carbohydrates: 20g, Protein: 30g
- Healthy Fats: 15g, Fiber: ~6g

Turkey and Avocado Lettuce Wraps

Ingredients:

8 ounces lean ground turkey

1 tablespoon olive oil

1 teaspoon cumin

1 teaspoon chili powder

Salt and pepper to taste

Iceberg lettuce leaves

1 avocado, sliced

1/4 cup salsa (sugar-free)

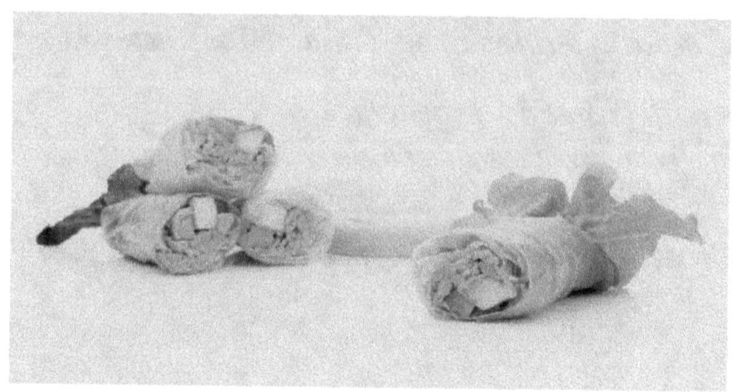

Preparation:

1. In a skillet, Warm your olive oil over medium heat.

2. Add ground turkey and heat until browned.

3. Add cumin, chili powder, salt, and pepper.

4. Wash and separate iceberg lettuce leaves.

5. Spoon the cooked turkey onto each lettuce leaf.

6. Top with sliced avocado and salsa.

7. Then wrap the lettuce around the filling and serve.

Cooking Time: 15 minutes

Serving: 2

Nutritional Value (Approximate):

- Calories: 300, Carbohydrates: 10g
- Protein: 20g, Healthy Fats: 18g, Fiber: 6g

Turkey and Vegetable Kebabs

Ingredients:

Eight ounces of turkey breast, sliced into cubes

1 zucchini, sliced

1 bell pepper, cut into pieces

Cherry tomatoes

2 tablespoons olive oil

1 teaspoon dried oregano

Salt and pepper to taste

Preparation:

1. In a bowl, combine turkey cubes, zucchini slices, bell pepper chunks, cherry tomatoes, olive oil, dried oregano, salt, and pepper.
2. Thread the vegetables and marinated turkey onto skewers.
3. Grill the kebabs until the turkey is fully cooked and the veggies are soft.
4. Serve hot.

Cooking Time: 15 minutes

Serving: 2 servings

Nutritional Value (Approximate):

- Calories: 320
- Carbohydrates: 15g, Protein: 25g
- Healthy Fats: 15g, Fiber: 5g

Spinach and Feta Stuffed Chicken Breast

Ingredients:

Two boneless, skinless chicken breasts

1 cup fresh spinach, chopped

1/4 cup feta cheese, crumbled

1 teaspoon olive oil

1 teaspoon minced garlic

Salt and pepper to taste

Lemon wedges for serving

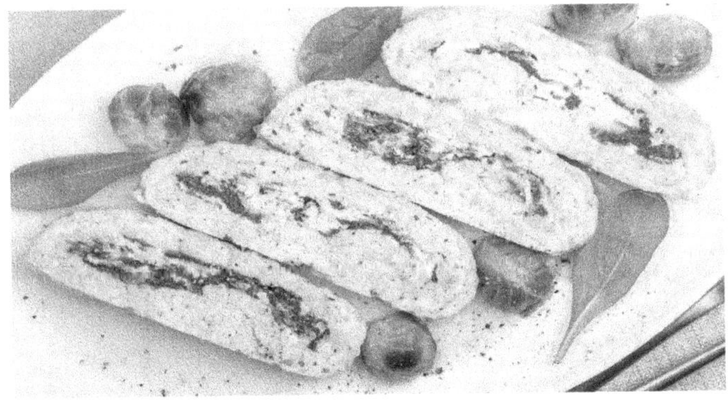

Preparation:

1. Set your oven to 375°F (190°C).

2. In a skillet, Warm your olive oil over medium heat.

3. Put minced garlic and chopped spinach, and sauté until spinach is wilted.

4. Butterfly each chicken breast and load with sautéed spinach and crumbled feta.

5. Add a little salt and pepper.

6. Secure the stuffed chicken breasts with toothpicks.

7. Put the filled chicken breasts in a baking dish.

8. Cook for 25 minutes or until the chicken is cooked through.

9. Remove toothpicks before serving.

10. Serve with lemon slices on the side.

Cooking Time:

Prep Time: 15 minutes

Bake Time: 25 minutes

Serving: 2 servings

Nutritional Value (Approximate):

- Calories: 300, Carbohydrates: 2g

- Protein: 40g, Healthy Fats: 12g

- Fiber: 1g

Quinoa Tabbouleh

Ingredients:

One cup of cooked quinoa

1 cup cherry tomatoes, diced

1 cucumber, diced

1/4 cup red onion, finely chopped

1/4 cup fresh parsley, chopped

2 tablespoons olive oil

2 teaspoons lemon juice

Salt and pepper to taste

Preparation:

1. In a bowl, add cooked quinoa, diced cherry tomatoes, cucumber, red onion, and chopped parsley.

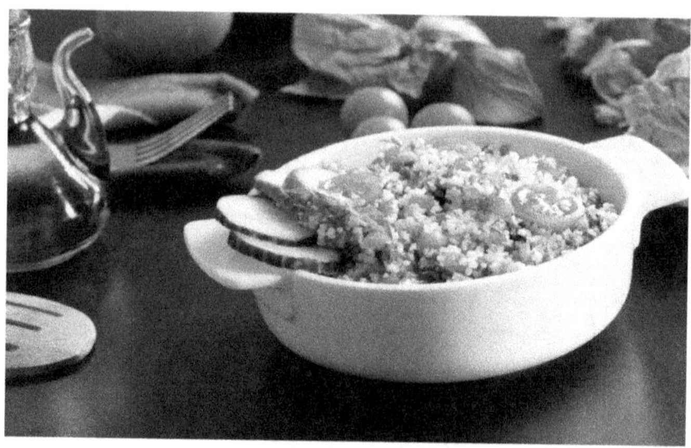

2. In a small bowl, whisk together lemon juice, olive oil, salt, and pepper to form a dressing.

3. Pour the dressing over the quinoa mixture and toss until fully incorporated.

4. keep in the refrigerator for at least 15 minutes before serving.

Cooking Time: 15 minutes

Serving: 2

Nutritional Value (Approximate):

- Calories: 250, Carbohydrates: 30g
- Protein: 5g, Healthy Fats: ~12g
- Fiber: ~4g

Lentil and Vegetable Soup

Ingredients:

1 cup dried green lentils, rinsed

1 onion, diced

2 carrots, diced

2 celery stalks, diced

3 cloves garlic, minced

6 cups vegetable broth

1 teaspoon ground cumin

1 teaspoon smoked paprika

Salt and pepper to taste

Fresh parsley for garnish (optional)

Preparation:

1. In a large pot, add lentils, diced onion, carrots, celery, and minced garlic.
2. Add vegetable broth, ground cumin, smoked paprika, salt, and pepper.
3. Bring to a boil, then decrease heat and simmer for 30 minutes or until lentils and vegetables are cooked.
4. Adjust seasoning as needed.
5. Decorate with fresh parsley before serving.

Cook Time: 30 minutes
Serving: 4 servings
Nutritional Value (Approximate):

- Calories: 300, Carbohydrates: 50g
- Protein: 15g, Healthy Fats: 2g

- Fiber: 20g

Grilled Chicken Salad with Balsamic Vinaigrette

Ingredients:

Four ounces of boneless, skinless chicken breast

4 cups mixed salad greens

1 cup cherry tomatoes, halved

1/2 cucumber, sliced

1/4 cup feta cheese, crumbled

2 tablespoons balsamic vinaigrette dressing (low-sugar)

Preparation:

1. Apply salt and pepper to the chicken breast.
2. Grill the chicken until fully done.

3. In a large bowl, combine salad leaves, cherry tomatoes, cucumber, and feta cheese.

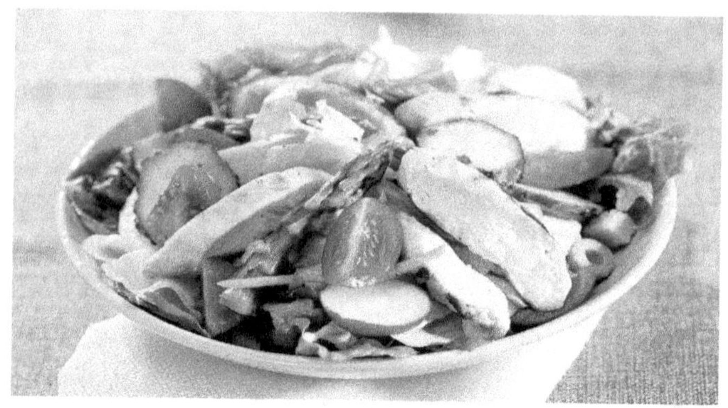

4. Slice grilled chicken and place on top of the salad.

5. Drizzle with balsamic vinaigrette dressing before serving.

Cooking Time: 15 minutes

Serving: 1 serving

Nutritional Value (Approximate):

- Calories: 350, Carbohydrates: 15g
- Protein: 30g, Healthy Fats: 15g

- Fiber: 5g

Quinoa Salad with Chickpeas and Veggies

Ingredients:

1/2 cup cooked quinoa

1/2 cup canned chickpeas, drained and rinsed

1/2 cup cherry tomatoes, halved

1/4 cup red bell pepper, chopped

1/4 cup cucumber, diced

2 tablespoons olive oil

1 tablespoon lemon juice

1 teaspoon dried oregano

Salt and pepper to taste

Preparation:

1. Cook quinoa according to package instructions.

2. In a large bowl, combine cooked quinoa, chickpeas, cherry tomatoes, red bell pepper, and cucumber.

3. In a small bowl, whisk together lemon juice, dried oregano, olive oil, salt, and pepper.

4. Pour the dressing over the quinoa mixture and toss until fully incorporated.

Cooking Time: 15 minutes

Serving: 1

Nutritional Value (Approximate):

- Calories: 300, Carbohydrates: 35g
- Protein: 10g, Healthy Fats: 15g, Fiber: 8g

Turkey and Vegetable Wrap with Whole-Grain Pita

Ingredients:

4 whole-grain pitas

1 pound lean ground turkey

1 tablespoon olive oil

1 small onion, coarsely chopped

2 cloves garlic, minced

1 teaspoon ground cumin

1 teaspoon paprika

1 teaspoon dried oregano

Salt and pepper to taste

1 cup cherry tomatoes, halved

1 cucumber, thinly sliced

1 cup shredded lettuce

1/2 cup Greek yogurt (low-fat or non-fat)

Fresh parsley for garnish (optional)

Preparation:

1. ***Cook Turkey Mixture:*** In a large skillet, heat olive oil over medium heat.

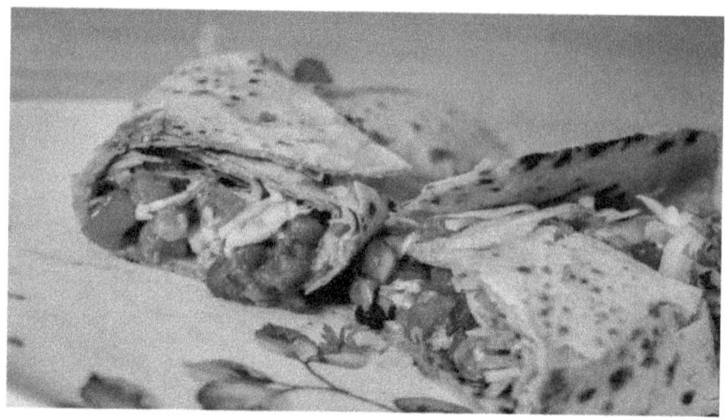

2. Pour in chopped onions and garlic, and sauté until softened.

3. Add ground turkey, cumin, paprika, oregano, salt, and pepper.

4. Cook until turkey is browned and cooked through.

5. ***Prepare Vegetables:*** While the turkey is cooking, prepare the vegetables.

6. Slice cherry tomatoes, cucumber, and shred the lettuce.

7. ***Assemble Wraps:*** Warm the whole-grain pitas in a dry skillet or microwave for a few seconds.

8. Spread a teaspoon of Greek yogurt onto each pita.

9. Add a portion of the cooked turkey mixture to the center of each pita.

10. Top with cherry tomatoes, cucumber slices, and shredded lettuce.

11. ***Garnish and Serve:*** Decorate with fresh parsley if preferred.

12. Fold the sides of the pita over the filling, creating a wrap.

13. Secure with toothpicks if necessary. Serve the Turkey and Vegetable Wraps immediately.

14. Pair with a side of raw veggies or a small salad for extra freshness.

Cooking Time: Prep Time: 15 minutes

Serving: 4

Nutritional Value (Approximate):

- Calories: 350
- Carbohydrates: 30g, Protein: 25g
- Healthy Fats: 12g, Fiber: 5g

Lentil and Vegetable Stir-Fry with Tofu

Ingredients:

1/2 cup cooked lentils

1/2 cup firm tofu, cubed

One cup of mixed veggies (broccoli, bell peppers, snap peas)

1 tablespoon low-sodium soy sauce

1 tablespoon olive oil

1 teaspoon minced garlic

1/2 teaspoon grated ginger

Sesame seeds for garnish (optional)

Preparation:

1. In a wok or skillet, Warm your olive oil over medium heat.
2. Put minced garlic and grated ginger, and sauté for a minute.
3. Add mixed vegetables and tofu cubes, and stir-fry until vegetables are soft.
4. Add cooked lentils and soy sauce, mix until well incorporated and heated through.
5. Decorate with sesame seeds if desired before serving.

Cooking Time:15 minutes

Serving: 1

Nutritional Value (Approximate):

- Calories: 320, Carbohydrates: 35g

- Protein: 18g, Healthy Fats: 12g
- Fiber: 10g

Salmon and Quinoa Bowl with Avocado

Ingredients:

2 salmon filets (approximately 6 oz each)

1 cup quinoa, washed

2 cups water or low-sodium chicken broth

1 tablespoon olive oil

1 teaspoon lemon zest

1 teaspoon dried dill

Salt and pepper to taste

1 avocado, sliced

1 cup cherry tomatoes, halved

1 cucumber, diced

2 cups mixed greens (spinach, arugula, or your preference)

Lemon wedges for serving

Preparation:

1. ***Cook Quinoa:*** In a medium saucepan, bring 2 cups of water or low-sodium chicken broth to a boil. Put your quinoa, reduce heat to low, cover, and simmer for about 15 minutes or until quinoa is cooked and water is absorbed. Fluff with a fork and set aside.

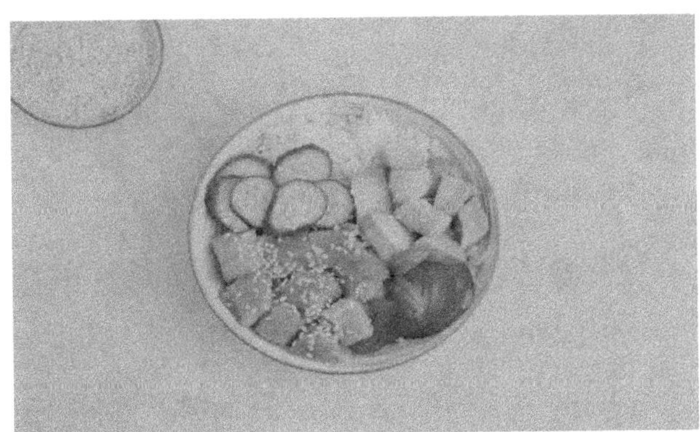

2. ***Prepare Salmon:*** Preheat the oven to 400°F (200°C). Place salmon filets on a baking pan lined with parchment

paper. Drizzle with olive oil and add lemon zest, dried dill, salt, and pepper.

3. Bake for 12-15 minutes or until the salmon is cooked through and flakes readily with a fork.

4. ***Assemble Bowls:*** Divide cooked quinoa among serving bowls. Top with cooked salmon filets, breaking them into large flakes. Arrange avocado slices, cherry tomatoes, cucumber, and mixed greens around the salmon.

5. ***Garnish and Serve:*** Garnish the bowl with more lemon zest, dill, and a wedge of lemon on the side. Drizzle with more olive oil if preferred.

6. Enjoy: Toss the ingredients together immediately before eating, ensuring the flavors combine well.

Cooking Time: 30 minutes

Serving: 2

Nutritional Value (Approximate):

- Calories: 500, Carbohydrates: 40g
- Protein: 30g, Healthy Fats: 25g
- Fiber: 10g

Mediterranean Chickpea Salad

Ingredients:

1 cup canned chickpeas, drained and rinsed

1/2 cup cherry tomatoes, halved

1/4 cup cucumber, diced

1/4 cup red bell pepper, chopped

2 tablespoons Kalamata olives, sliced

1/4 cup feta cheese, crumbled

2 tablespoons olive oil

1 tablespoon red wine vinegar

1 teaspoon dried oregano

Salt and pepper to taste

Preparation Time: 5 minutes

Serving: 1

Nutritional Value (Approximate):

- Calories: 320, Carbohydrates: 30g
- Protein: 10g, Healthy Fats: 18g
- Fiber: 8g

Preparation:

1. In a large bowl, add chickpeas, cherry tomatoes, cucumber, red bell pepper, olives, and feta cheese.
2. In a small bowl, whisk together olive oil, red wine vinegar, dried oregano, salt, and pepper.

3. Pour the dressing over the chickpea mixture and toss until well incorporated.

Turkey and Vegetable Stir-Fry with Brown Rice

Ingredients:

Four ounces of lean ground turkey

One cup of mixed veggies (broccoli, carrots, bell peppers)

1/2 cup cooked brown rice

1 tablespoon low-sodium soy sauce

1 tablespoon olive oil

1 teaspoon minced garlic

1/2 teaspoon grated ginger

Sesame seeds for garnish (optional)

Preparation:

1. In a skillet, Warm your olive oil over medium heat.

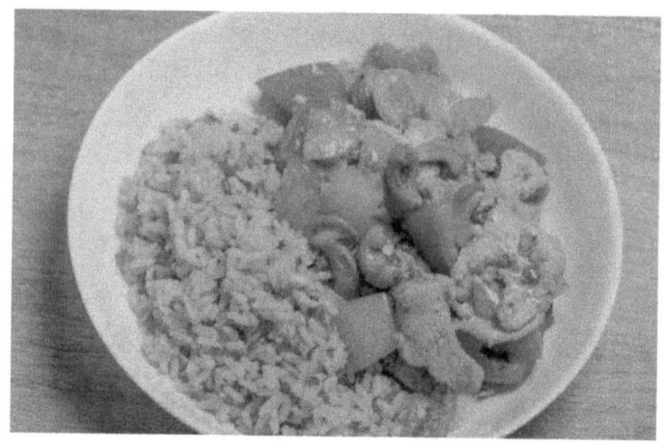

2. Put minced garlic and grated ginger, and sauté for a minute.

3. Add ground turkey and heat until browned.

4. Add mixed vegetables and continue to stir-fry until vegetables are cooked.

5. Add cooked brown rice and soy sauce, and mix until thoroughly blended and heated through.

6. Garnish with sesame seeds if desired before serving.

Cooking Time: 15 minutes

Serving: 1

Nutritional Value (Approximate):

- Calories: 340 Carbohydrates: 35g

- Protein: 20g, Healthy Fats: 15g

- Fiber: 6g

Caprese Quinoa Bowl

Ingredients:

1/2 cup cooked quinoa

1/2 cup cherry tomatoes, halved

1/4 cup fresh mozzarella, diced

1/4 cup fresh basil leaves, torn

1 tablespoon balsamic glaze

1 tablespoon olive oil

Salt and pepper to taste

Preparation:

1. Cook quinoa according to package instructions.

2. Cook quinoa, Cherry tomatoes, fresh mozzarella, and torn basil leaves, all should be combined in a bowl.

3. Drizzle with balsamic glaze and olive oil.

4. Add salt and pepper, and mix until thoroughly incorporated.

5. Serve warm.

Cooking Time: 15 minutes

Serving: 1

Nutritional Value (Approximate):

- Calories: 300
- Carbohydrates: 25g, Protein: 12g
- Healthy Fats: 15g, Fiber: 4g

Chicken and Vegetable Quinoa Stir-Fry

Ingredients:

Four oz boneless, skinless chicken breast, thinly sliced

half cup cooked quinoa

One cup of mixed veggies (broccoli, snap peas, carrots)

1 tablespoon low-sodium soy sauce

1 tablespoon sesame oil

1 teaspoon minced garlic

1/2 teaspoon grated ginger

Green onions for garnish (optional)

Preparation:

1. In a wok or skillet, Warm your sesame oil over medium heat.

2. Put the minced garlic and grated ginger, and sauté for a minute.

3. Add thinly sliced chicken and heat until browned.

4. Add mixed vegetables and continue to stir-fry until vegetables are cooked.

5. Add cooked quinoa and soy sauce, and mix until well blended and heated through.

6. Garnish with green onions if desired.

Cooking Time: 15 minutes

Serving: 1

Nutritional Value (Approximate):

- Calories: 330
- Carbohydrates: 30g, Protein: 25g
- Healthy Fats: 12g, Fiber: 5g

Mushroom and Spinach Whole-Grain Wrap

Ingredients:

1 whole-grain wrap

1 cup mushrooms, sliced

1 cup fresh spinach leaves

1/4 cup red bell pepper, thinly sliced

2 tablespoons hummus

1 tablespoon olive oil

Salt and pepper to taste

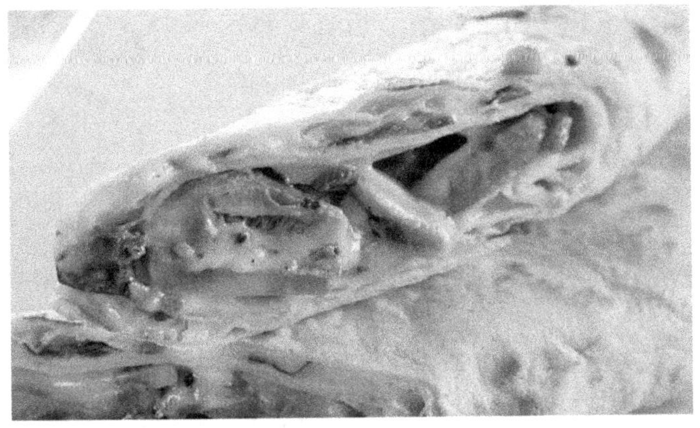

Preparation:

1. In a skillet, Warm your olive oil over medium heat.

2. Add sliced mushrooms and red bell pepper, and sauté until mushrooms are browned.

3. Add fresh spinach leaves and simmer until wilted.

4. Warm the whole-grain wrap.

5. Extend the hummus over the wrap and layer the cooked vegetables.

6. Season with salt and pepper.

7. Fold the wrap and serve.

Cooking Time: 10 minutes

Serving: 1

Nutritional Value (Approximate):

- Calories: 290, Carbohydrates: 30g
- Protein: 10g, Healthy Fats: 15g
- Fiber: ~6g

Dinner recipes:

Baked Cod with Lemon and Dill

Ingredients:

2 cod filets (6 oz each)

1 lemon, sliced

2 tablespoons fresh dill, chopped

1 tablespoon olive oil

Salt and pepper to taste

Preparation:

1. Preheat your oven to 375°F (190°C).

2. Place cod filets on a baking sheet.

3. Pour olive oil and add a little salt and pepper.

4. Arrange lemon slices over top and sprinkle with minced dill.

5. Bake for 15 minutes or until the cod is flaky and cooked through.

6. Serve with more lemon slices.

Cooking Time: 15 minutes

Serving: 2

Nutritional Value (Approximate):

- Calories: 200, Carbohydrates: 2g

- Protein: 40g, Healthy Fats: 5g
- Fiber: 1g

Beef Stir-Fry with Broccoli, Bell Peppers, and Snap Peas

Ingredients:

8 lb beef sirloin, thinly sliced

2 cups broccoli florets

1 bell pepper, thinly sliced

1 cup snap peas, ends cut

2 teaspoons low-sodium soy sauce

1 tablespoon sesame oil

1 teaspoon minced garlic

1/2 teaspoon grated ginger

Green onions for garnish (optional)

Preparation:

1. In a wok or skillet, heat sesame oil over medium heat.

2. Add chopped meat, minced garlic, and grated ginger. Stir-fry until beef is browned.

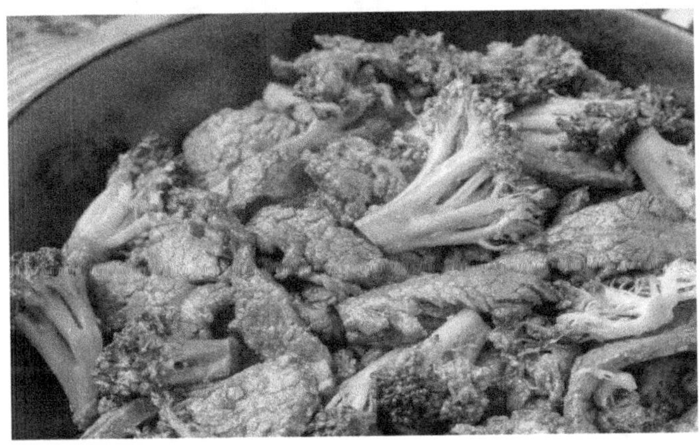

3. Add broccoli, bell pepper, and snap peas. Stir-fry until vegetables are soft.

4. Pour in soy sauce and mix until thoroughly incorporated and cooked through.

5. Decorate with green onions if desired before serving.

Cooking Time: 15 minutes

Serving: 2

Nutritional Value (Approximate):

- Calories: 350, Carbohydrates: 15g

- Protein: 25g, Healthy Fats: 18g

- Fiber: 6g

Baked Tilapia with Garlic and Herbs

Ingredients:

2 tilapia filets (6 oz each)

2 tablespoons olive oil

2 cloves garlic, minced

1 tablespoon fresh parsley, chopped

1 teaspoon dried thyme

Salt and pepper to taste

Lemon wedges for serving

Preparation:

1. Preheat the oven to 400°F (200°C).

2. Place tilapia filets on a baking sheet.

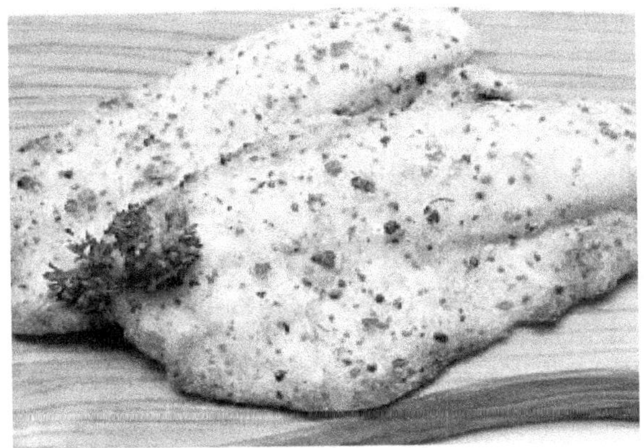

3. Drizzle with olive oil and sprinkle with minced garlic, chopped parsley, dried thyme, salt, and pepper.

4. Bake for 12 minutes or until the tilapia is cooked through.

5. Serve with lemon slices on the side.

Cooking Time: 15 minutes

Serving: 2

Nutritional Value (Approximate):

- Calories: 180
- Carbohydrates: 1g, Protein: 25g

- Healthy Fats: 9g, Fiber: 0g

Grilled Salmon with Honey-Mustard Glaze

Ingredients:

2 salmon filets (6 oz each)

2 teaspoons Dijon mustard

1 tablespoon honey

1 tablespoon olive oil

1 teaspoon lemon juice

Salt and pepper to taste

Preparation:

1. Preheat the grill to medium-high heat.

2. In a bowl, whisk together Dijon mustard, honey, olive oil, lemon juice, salt, and pepper.

3. Brush the honey-mustard glaze over the salmon filets.

4. Grill salmon for roughly 4-5 minutes per side or until done through.

5. Decorate with fresh dill before serving. (Fresh dill for garnish (optional)

Cooking Time (Preparation): 10 minutes

Grilling Time: 10 minutes

Serving: 2

Nutritional Value (Approximate):

- Calories: 350

- Carbohydrates: 8g, Protein: 30g

- Healthy Fats: 20g, Fiber: ~0g

Beef and Vegetable Kebabs with Soy-Ginger Marinade

Ingredients:

8 ounces beef sirloin, sliced into cubes

1 zucchini, sliced

1 bell pepper, cut into pieces

1 red onion, cut into wedges

1 cup cherry tomatoes

1/4 cup low-sodium soy sauce

2 tablespoons olive oil

1 tablespoon rice vinegar

1 tablespoon honey

1 teaspoon minced ginger

1 teaspoon minced garlic

Sesame seeds for garnish (optional)

Preparation:

1. In a bowl, whisk together soy sauce, olive oil, rice vinegar, honey, minced ginger, and minced garlic.

2. Thread beef pieces, zucchini slices, bell pepper chunks, red onion wedges, and cherry tomatoes onto skewers.

3. Place the skewers in a shallow dish and brush with the soy-ginger marinade.

4. Keep it to marinate for at least 15 minutes.

5. Preheat the grill to medium-high heat.

6. Grill kebabs for around 5-7 minutes per side or until the beef is cooked to your preference.

7. Decorate with sesame seeds before serving.

Cooking Time: 20 minutes

Serving: 2

Nutritional Value (Approximate):
- Calories: 400, Carbohydrates: 20g
- Protein: 25g, Healthy Fats: 20g
- Fiber: 4g

Baked Salmon with Asparagus and Quinoa

Ingredients:

2 salmon filets (6 oz each)

1 bunch asparagus, trimmed

1 cup cooked quinoa

1 tablespoon olive oil

1 teaspoon lemon zest

1 teaspoon dried dill

Salt and pepper to taste

Lemon wedges for serving

Preparation:

1. Preheat your oven to 400°F (200°C).

2. Place salmon filets and trimmed asparagus on a baking sheet.

3. Drizzle with olive oil and sprinkle with lemon zest, dried dill, salt, and pepper.

4. Cook for 15 minutes or until salmon is cooked through.

5. Serve over a bed of cooked quinoa.

6. Decorate with lemon wedges.

Cooking Time: 20 minutes

Serving: 2

Nutritional Value (Approximate):

- Calories: 400, Carbohydrates: 25g
- Protein: 30g, Healthy Fats: 20g
- Fiber: 5g

Vegetarian Eggplant and Chickpea Stew

Ingredients:

1 large eggplant, diced

Rinsed and drained 1 can (15 oz) of chickpeas

1 onion, diced

2 cloves garlic, minced

1 can (14 oz) diced tomatoes

1 teaspoon cumin

1 teaspoon paprika

1/2 teaspoon cinnamon

2 cups vegetable broth

Salt and pepper to taste

Fresh parsley for garnish (optional)

1 tablespoon olive oil

Preparation:

1. In a pot, Warm your olive oil over medium heat.

2. Put diced onion and garlic, and sauté until softened.

3. Add diced eggplant and cook until lightly browned.

4. Stir in chickpeas, diced tomatoes, cumin, paprika, cinnamon, salt, and pepper.

5. Pour in vegetable broth, bring to a simmer, and let it cook for 20-25 minutes.

6. Decorate with fresh parsley before serving.

Cooking Time: 30 minutes

Serving: 4

Nutritional Value (Approximate):

- Calories: 330
- Carbohydrates: 45g, Protein: 12g
- Healthy Fats: 10g, Fiber: 15g

Shrimp and Vegetable Stir-Fry with Cauliflower Rice

Ingredients:

8 oz shrimp, peeled and deveined

2 cups cauliflower rice

1 cup broccoli florets

1/2 cup snap peas

1 carrot, julienned

1 tablespoon low-sodium soy sauce

1 tablespoon sesame oil

1 teaspoon minced garlic

1/2 teaspoon grated ginger

Green onions for garnish (optional)

Preparation:

1. In a wok or skillet, Warm your sesame oil over medium heat.

2. Add shrimp, minced garlic, and grated ginger. Stir-fry until the shrimp turns pink.

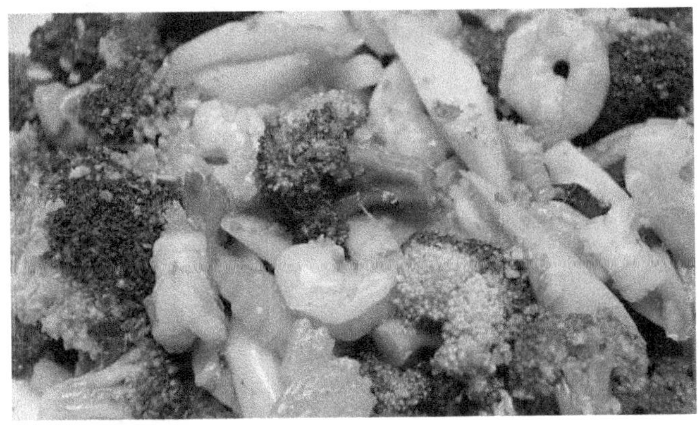

3. Add broccoli, snap peas, and julienned carrot. Stir-fry until vegetables are tender.

4. Stir in cauliflower rice and soy sauce, toss until well combined and heated through.

5. Decorate with green onions if desired.

Cooking Time: 15 minutes

Serving: 2

Nutritional Value (Approximate):

- Calories: 320
- Carbohydrates: 20g, Protein: 25g
- Healthy Fats: 15g, Fiber: 8g

Mushroom and Spinach Stuffed Bell Peppers

Ingredients:

Two bell peppers, halved and seeds removed

1 cup quinoa, cooked

1 cup mushrooms, chopped

2 cups fresh spinach, chopped

Half cup of feta cheese, crumbled

1 teaspoon olive oil

1 teaspoon Italian seasoning

Salt and pepper to taste

Preparation:

1. Set your oven to 375°F (190°C).

2. In a skillet, Warm your olive oil over medium heat.

3. Add chopped mushrooms and cook until softened.

4. Stir in chopped spinach and allow to cook until wilted.

5. In a bowl, combine cooked quinoa, mushroom-spinach mixture, and crumbled feta.

6. Stuffed bell pepper halves with the quinoa mixture.

7. Place stuffed peppers in a baking dish and bake for 20 minutes or until peppers are tender.

Cooking Time: 25 minutes

Serving: 4

Nutritional Value (Approximate):

- Calories: 350, Carbohydrates: 35g

- Protein: 12g, Healthy Fats: 15g
- Fiber: 8g

Baked Chicken Breast with Roasted Vegetables

Ingredients:

2 boneless, skinless chicken breasts

Two cups of mixed vegetables (zucchini, bell peppers, cherry tomatoes)

1 tablespoon olive oil

1 teaspoon dried rosemary

1 teaspoon garlic powder

Salt and pepper to taste

Lemon wedges for serving

Preparation:

1. Set your oven to 400°F (200°C).
2. Place chicken breasts and mixed vegetables on a baking sheet.

3. Drizzle with olive oil and sprinkle with dried rosemary, garlic powder, salt, and pepper.

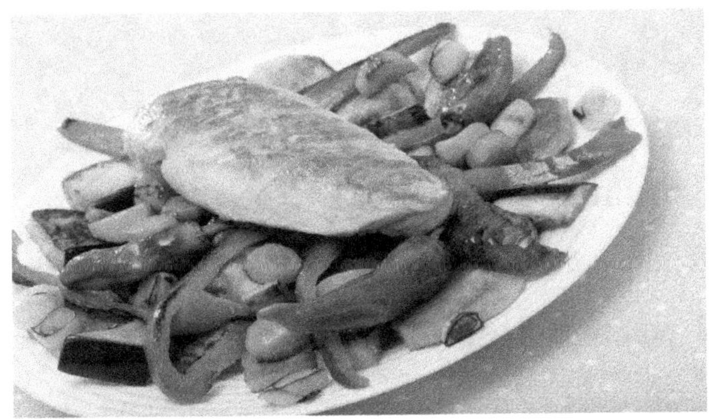

4. Bake for 25 minutes or until chicken is cooked through and vegetables are tender.

5. Serve with lemon wedges on the side.

Cooking Time: 30 minutes

Serving: 2

Nutritional Value (Approximate):

- Calories: 350, Carbohydrates: 15g

- Protein: 30g, Healthy Fats: 15g

- Fiber: 5g

Vegetarian Cauliflower and Chickpea Curry

Ingredients:

1 cauliflower, cut into florets

Rinse and drained 1 can (15 oz) chickpeas

1 onion, finely chopped

2 cloves garlic, minced

1 can (14 oz) diced tomatoes

1 can (14 oz) coconut milk (light)

2 tablespoons curry powder

1 teaspoon ground cumin

1 teaspoon ground coriander

Salt and pepper to taste

Fresh cilantro for garnish (optional)

1 tablespoon olive oil

Preparation:

1. In a large pot, Heat your olive oil over medium heat.

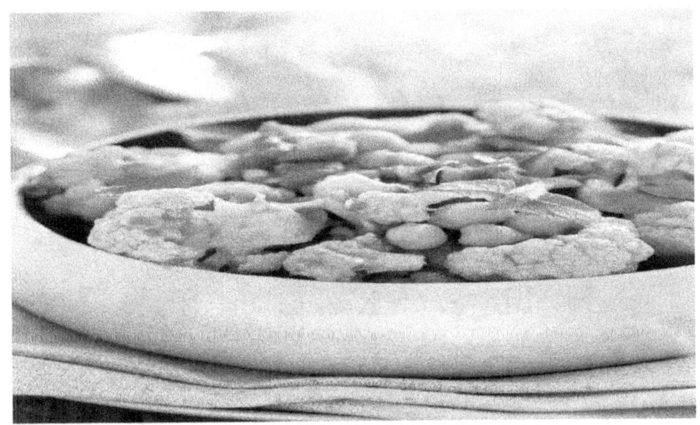

2. Add chopped onion and garlic, and sauté until softened.

3. Add cauliflower florets, chickpeas, diced tomatoes, coconut milk, curry powder, ground cumin, ground coriander, salt, and pepper.

4. Bring to a simmer and allow to cook for 25 minutes or until the cauliflower is tender.

5. Decorate with fresh cilantro before serving.

Cooking Time: 25 minutes

Serving: 4

Nutritional Value (Approximate):

- Calories: 380
- Carbohydrates: 45g, Protein: 15g
- Healthy Fats: 15g, Fiber: 15g

Tuna Melts with Avocado and Whole Wheat English Muffins

Ingredients:

1 can (5 oz) tuna, drained

1 tablespoon mayonnaise (light or reduced-fat)

1 tablespoon Dijon mustard

1 tablespoon chopped fresh dill

1/4 cup chopped red onion

1/4 avocado, thinly sliced

2 whole wheat English muffins, toasted

1 piece of low-fat Swiss cheese per sandwich

Preparation:

1. In a bowl, combine tuna, mayonnaise, Dijon mustard, dill, and red onion.

2. Spread the mixture onto one-half of each toasted English muffin.

3. Top with avocado slices and cheese.

4. Broil for 2-3 minutes, or until the cheese is melted and slightly browned.

Cooking Time: 5 minutes

Serving: 2

Nutritional Value (Per serving):

- Calories: 350

- Carbohydrates: 30g

- Protein: 25g, healthy Fat: 15g

Shrimp Scampi with Zucchini Noodles and Whole Wheat Pasta

Ingredients:

1/2 lb big shrimp, peeled and deveined

1 tablespoon olive oil

2 cloves garlic, minced

1/4 cup dry white wine

1/4 cup chicken broth

1 tablespoon lemon juice

1/4 teaspoon dried oregano

1/8 teaspoon red pepper flakes (optional)

1 medium zucchini, spiralized

1/2 cup cooked whole wheat pasta

Fresh parsley, chopped

Preparation:

1. Warm your olive oil in a pan over
   medium heat. Put garlic and heat for
   30 seconds.

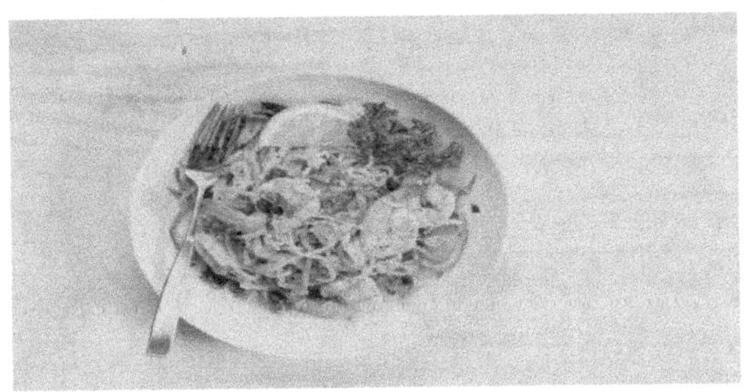

2. Add shrimp and heat until pink and
   opaque, about 2-3 minutes per side.
3. Deglaze the pan with white wine,
   scraping up any browned bits.
4. Add chickcn broth, lemon juice,
   oregano, and red pepper flakes (if
   using). Bring to a simmer and cook
   for 2 minutes.
5. Add zucchini noodles and cook until
   tender-crisp, about 2-3 minutes.

6. Stir in cooked spaghetti and heat through.

7. Serve garnished with fresh parsley.

Cooking Time: 10 minutes

Serving: 2

Nutritional Value (Per serving):

- Calories: 450
- Carbohydrates: 40g , Protein: 35g

Mediterranean Turkey Meatballs with Zucchini Noodles

Ingredients:

1 pound ground turkey breast

1/2 cup sliced onion

1/4 cup chopped fresh parsley

1 tablespoon olive oil

1 teaspoon dried oregano

1/2 teaspoon salt

1/4 teaspoon black pepper

2 medium zucchini, spiralized

Preparation:

1. Preheat your oven to 375°F (190°C).

2. In a bowl, combine turkey, onion, parsley, olive oil, oregano, salt, and pepper. Mix well. Form into little meatballs.

3. Leave it to bake for 20-25 minutes, or until cooked through.

4. Meanwhile, spiralize zucchini into noodles.

5. While you are baking the meatballs warm your pan with a drizzle of olive oil. Sauté zucchini noodles until slightly tender.

6. Serve meatballs over zucchini noodles.

Serving: 4

Nutritional Value(Per serving):

- Calories: 300

- Carbohydrates: 15g , Protein: 30g

- Fat: 10g

Chapter 5: Super Seafoods

Pan-seared cod with Lemon and Herb Butter

Ingredients:

2 cod filets (6 oz each)

2 tablespoons unsalted butter

1 tablespoon fresh lemon juice

1 teaspoon fresh parsley, chopped

1 teaspoon fresh thyme, diced

Salt and pepper to taste

Preparation:

1. Apply salt and pepper to the cod filets.
2. In a skillet, warm your butter over medium-high heat.

3. Add cod filets and sear for 4 minutes per side or until the fish is opaque and flakes readily.

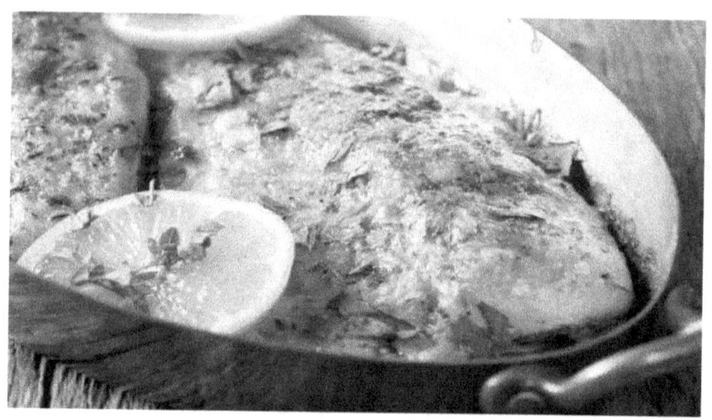

4. In the last minute of cooking, add lemon juice, chopped parsley, and chopped thyme to the skillet.

5. Spoon the herb butter over the fish filets before serving.

Cooking Time: 15 minutes

Serving: 2

Nutritional Value (Approximate):

- Calories: 250

- Carbohydrates: 2g, Protein: 30g

- Healthy Fats: 15g, Fiber: 0g

Salmon and Avocado Salad

Ingredients:

2 salmon filets (6 oz each)

4 cups mixed salad greens

1 avocado, sliced

1/4 cup cherry tomatoes, halved

2 tablespoons olive oil

1 tablespoon balsamic vinegar

1 teaspoon Dijon mustard

Salt and pepper to taste

Preparation:

1. Preheat your grill to medium-high heat.
2. Season salmon filets with salt and pepper.

3. Grill salmon for about 4-5 minutes per side or until the fish is cooked through.

4. In a large bowl, toss Cherry Tomatoes, mixed salad greens, and sliced avocado.

5. In a small bowl, whisk together pepper, salt, Dijon mustard, olive oil, and balsamic vinegar.

6. Drizzle the dressing over the salad and top with cooked salmon.

Cooking Time: 20 minutes

Serving: 2

Nutritional Value (Approximate):

- Calories: 400
- Carbohydrates: 15g, Protein: 30g
- Healthy Fats: 25g, Fiber: 7g

Tuna and White Bean Salad

Ingredients:

One can (5 oz) of tuna in water, drained

Rinsed and drained 1 can (15 oz) white beans

1 cup cherry tomatoes, halved

1/4 cup red onion, fincly choppcd

2 tablespoons fresh parsley, chopped

2 tablespoons olive oil

1 tablespoon red wine vinegar

Salt and pepper to taste

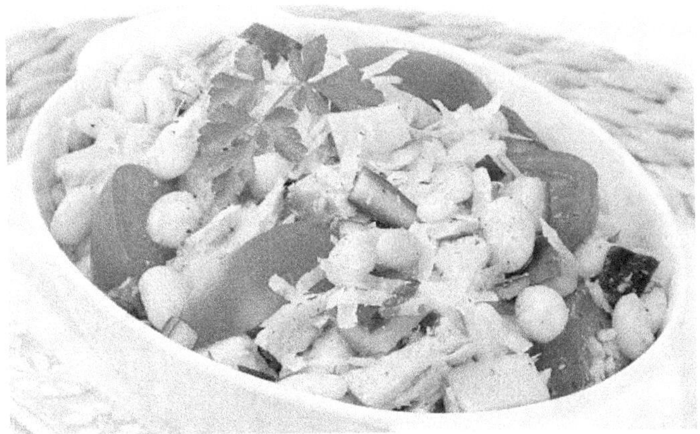

Preparation:

1. In a bowl, add tuna, white beans, cherry tomatoes, red onion, and fresh parsley.
2. In a small bowl, whisk together red wine vinegar, olive oil, salt, and pepper to form a dressing.
3. Add the dressing over the tuna and white bean mixture.
4. Toss until fully incorporated and refrigerate for at least 15 minutes before serving.

Serving: 2

Nutritional Value (Approximate):

- Calories: 300
- Carbohydrates: 30g, Protein: 20g
- Healthy Fats: 12g, Fiber: 10g

Mediterranean Shrimp and Quinoa Bowl

Ingredients:

Eight ounces of shrimp peeled and deveined

1 cup cooked quinoa

1/2 cup cucumber, diced

1/2 cup cherry tomatoes, halved

1/4 cup Kalamata olives, sliced

2 tablespoons feta cheese, crumbled

Two tablespoons of olive oil

1 tablespoon lemon juice

1 teaspoon dried oregano

Salt and pepper to taste

Preparation:

1. In a skillet, Warm your olive oil over medium heat.

2. Add prawns and cook until pink and opaque.

3. In a bowl, add cooked quinoa, chopped cucumber, cherry tomatoes, sliced Kalamata olives, and feta cheese.

4. In a small bowl, stir together lemon juice, dried oregano, salt, and pepper.

5. Pour the dressing over the quinoa mixture and top with cooked shrimp.

Cooking Time: 10 minutes

Serving: 2

Nutritional Value (Approximate):

- Calories: 350, Carbohydrates: 25g
- Protein: 25g
- Healthy Fats: 18g, Fiber: 5g

Baked Lemon Garlic Butter Scallops

Ingredients:

1 pound sea scallops

2 tablespoons unsalted butter,

melted 2 teaspoons of fresh lemon juice

2 cloves garlic, minced

1 tablespoon fresh parsley, chopped

Salt and pepper to taste

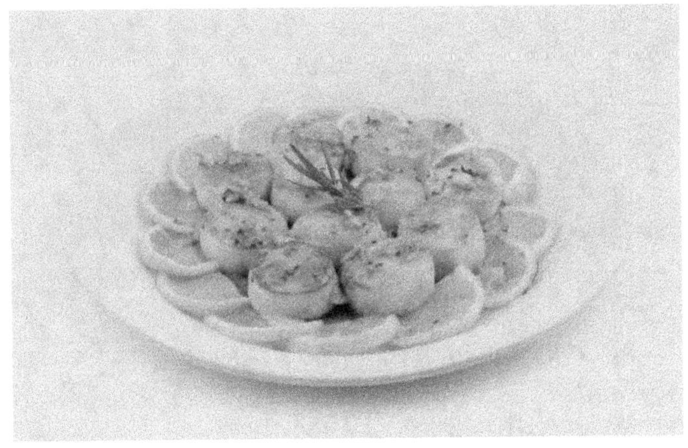

Preparation:

1. Set your oven to 375°F (190°C).

2. Pat dry scallops with a paper towel
    and set them in a baking dish.

3. In a bowl, mix melted butter, lemon juice, minced garlic, chopped parsley, salt, and pepper.

4. Pour the mixture over the scallops.

5. Bake for 12 minutes or until the scallops are opaque and cooked

Cooking Time: 20 minutes

Serving: 2

Nutritional Value (Approximate):

- Calories: 250

- Carbohydrates: 6g, Protein: 30g

- Healthy Fats: 12g, Fiber: 1g

Lemon Herb Grilled Tuna Steaks

Ingredients:

2 tuna steaks (6 oz each)

2 tablespoons olive oil

1 tablespoon fresh lemon juice

1 teaspoon fresh thyme, diced

1 teaspoon fresh rosemary, chopped

1 clove garlic, minced

Salt and pepper to taste

Preparation:

1. In a bowl, mix olive oil, fresh lemon juice, chopped thyme, chopped rosemary, minced garlic, salt, and pepper.

2. Marinate the tuna steaks in the marinade for at least 15 minutes.

3. Preheat your grill to medium-high heat.

4. Grill tuna steaks for about 3-4 minutes per side or until the tuna is

seared on the outside but still pink in
the center.

5. Serve with more lemon wedges if
desired.

Cooking Time: 15 minutes

Serving: 2

Nutritional Value (Approximate):

- Calories: 300
- Carbohydrates: 0g, Protein: 40g
- Healthy Fats: 15g, Fiber: 0g

Chapter 6: Rice and pasta

Brown Rice and Vegetable Pilaf

Ingredients:

1 cup brown rice, uncooked

2 cups mixed veggies (peas, carrots, corn), diced

1/4 cup almonds, chopped

1 tablespoon olive oil

1 teaspoon cumin

1 teaspoon turmeric

2 cups vegetable broth (low-sodium)

Salt and pepper to taste

Fresh cilantro for garnish (optional)

Preparation:

1. In a saucepan, Warm your olive oil over medium heat.

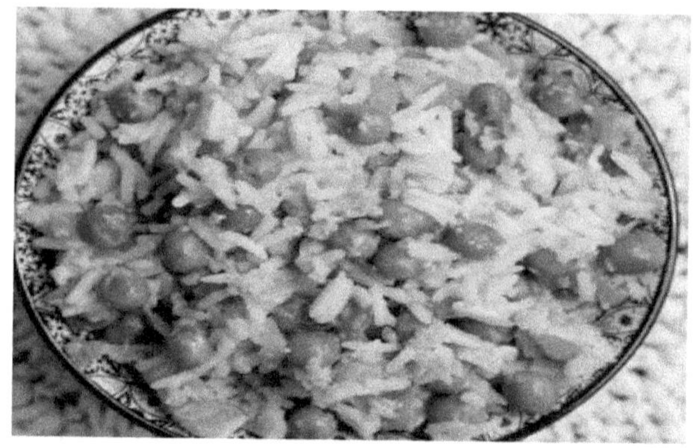

2. Add brown rice, sliced almonds, cumin, and turmeric. Toast for 2-3 minutes.

3. Add diced mixed vegetables and sauté for an additional 5 minutes.

4. Pour in vegetable broth, bring to a boil, then reduce heat, cover, and simmer for 30-35 minutes or until rice is cooked.

5. Fluff the rice with a fork, season with salt and pepper, then garnish with fresh cilantro if preferred.

Cooking Time: 40 minutes

Serving: 2

Nutritional Value (Approximate):

- Calories: 320
- Carbohydrates: 50g, Protein: 8g
- Healthy Fats: 10g, Fiber: 7g

Whole Wheat Pasta with Tomato and Spinach Sauce

Ingredients:

Eight oz whole wheat pasta

One can (14 oz) chopped tomatoes

2 cups fresh spinach

Two tablespoons of olive oil

2 cloves garlic, minced

1 teaspoon dried basil

1 teaspoon dried oregano

Salt and pepper to taste

Grated Parmesan cheese for garnish (optional)

Preparation:

1. The whole wheat pasta should be cooked according to package instructions.

2. In a large saucepan, Warm your olive oil over medium heat.

3. Put minced garlic and sauté until fragrant.

4. Put diced tomatoes, dried basil, dried oregano, salt, and pepper. Simmer for 10 minutes.

5. Stir in fresh spinach and cook until wilted.

6. Toss the cooked pasta in the tomato and spinach sauce.

7. Decorate with grated Parmesan cheese if preferred.

Cooking Time: 15 minutes

Serving: 2

Nutritional Value (Approximate):

- Calories: 300
- Carbohydrates: 45g, Protein: 10g
- Healthy Fats: 10g, Fiber: ~8g

Lemon Garlic Shrimp with Brown Rice

Ingredients:

Eight ounces of shrimp, peeled and deveined

1 cup brown rice, uncooked

2 tablespoons olive oil

2 cloves garlic, minced

Zest and juice of 1 lemon

1 teaspoon dried thyme

Salt and pepper to taste

Fresh parsley for garnish (optional)

Preparation:

1. The brown rice should be cooked according to package instructions.

2. In a skillet, Warm your olive oil over medium heat.

3. Put minced garlic and sauté until fragrant.

4. Put shrimp, lemon zest, lemon juice, dried thyme, salt, and pepper. Then allow to cook until shrimp is pink and opaque.

5. Serve the lemon garlic shrimp over cooked brown rice.

6. Garnish with fresh parsley if preferred.

Cooking Time: 20 minutes

Serving: 2

Nutritional Value (Approximate):

- Calories: 350
- Carbohydrates: 40g, Protein: 20g
- Healthy Fats: 12g, Fiber: 4g

Vegetarian Pasta Primavera

Ingredients:

Eight oz whole wheat pasta

2 cups mixed veggies (zucchini, cherry tomatoes, bell peppers), sliced

2 tablespoons olive oil

2 cloves garlic, minced

1 teaspoon dried Italian seasoning

Salt and pepper to taste

Grated Parmesan cheese for garnish (optional)

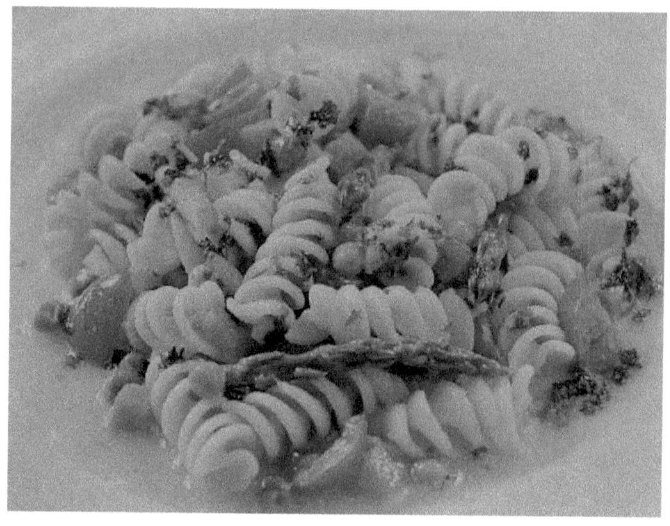

Preparation:

1. The whole wheat pasta should be cooked according to package instructions.

2. In a large skillet, heat your olive oil over medium heat.

3. Add minced garlic and sauté until fragrant.

4. Add sliced vegetables and dry Italian seasoning. Cook until vegetables are tender-crisp.

5. Toss the cooked spaghetti with the veggie mixture.

6. Add salt and pepper, then sprinkle with grated Parmesan cheese if preferred.

Cooking Time: 15 minutes

Serving: 2

Nutritional Value (Approximate):

- Calories: 320
- Carbohydrates: 50g, Protein: 10g
- Healthy Fats: 10g, Fiber: 8g

Mushroom and Spinach Risotto

Ingredients:

1 cup Arborio rice

1/2 cup white wine (optional)

2 cups mushrooms, sliced

2 cups fresh spinach, chopped

1 onion, finely chopped

4 cups vegetable broth (low-sodium)

2 tablespoons olive oil

1/4 cup grated Parmesan cheese

Salt and pepper to taste

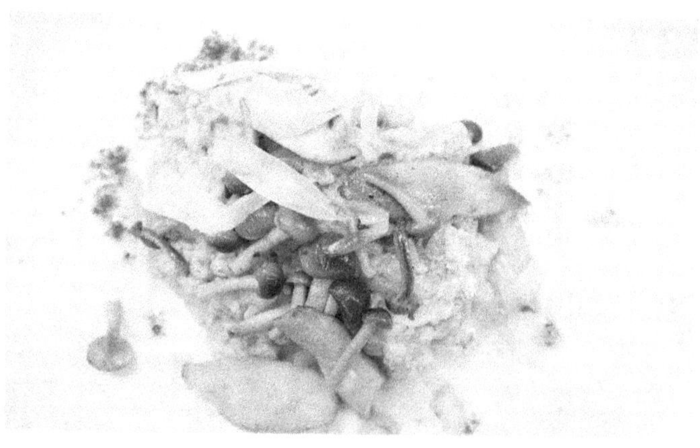

Preparation:

1. In a saucepan, heat vegetable broth and keep it warm over low heat.

2. In a separate big skillet, heat olive oil over medium heat.

3. Add chopped onion and sauté until softened.

4. Add Arborio rice and swirl to coat with oil until slightly transparent.

5. If using, pour in white wine and simmer until largely evaporated.

6. Begin adding warm vegetable broth one ladle at a time, stirring regularly and letting the liquid be absorbed before adding more.

7. Stir and add sliced mushrooms and chopped spinach halfway through the cooking procedure.

8. Continue until the rice is creamy and cooked to your taste.

9. Stir in grated Parmesan cheese and add a little salt and pepper.

Cooking Time: 30 Minutes

Serving: 2

Nutritional Value (Approximate):

- Calories: 380

- Carbohydrates: 50g, Protein: ~8g

- Healthy Fats: 14g, Fiber: 5g

Spaghetti Squash with Tomato Basil Sauce

Ingredients:

1 medium-sized spaghetti squash

1 can (14 oz) chopped tomatoes

2 cloves garlic, minced

2 tablespoons olive oil

1 teaspoon dried basil

1/2 teaspoon dried oregano

Salt and pepper to taste

Grated Pecorino Romano cheese for garnish (optional)

Preparation:

1. Set your oven to 375°F (190°C).

2. Pieces the spaghetti squash in half lengthwise and scoop out the seeds.

3. Place the squash halves on a baking pan, and cut side up.

4. Drizzle with olive oil and season with minced garlic, dried basil, dried oregano, salt, and pepper.

5. Roast in the oven for 45 minutes or until the squash is soft. Then use a fork to scrape the squash into spaghetti-like strands.

6. In a saucepan, cook diced tomatoes until warmed.

7. Serve the tomato basil sauce over the spaghetti squash.

8. Garnish with shredded Pecorino Romano cheese if preferred.

Cooking Time: 50 minutes

Serving: 2

Nutritional Value (Approximate):

- Calories: 250
- Carbohydrates: 30g, Protein: 4g
- Healthy Fats: 15g, Fiber: 7g

Chapter 7: Snacks:

Vegetable Sticks with Hummus

Ingredients:

1 cup carrot sticks

1 cup cucumber sticks

1/2 cup cherry tomatoes

1/4 cup hummus

Preparation:

1. Arrange carrot sticks, cucumber sticks, and cherry tomatoes on a platter.
2. Serve with a side of hummus for dipping.
3. Enjoy this crispy and delicious snack.

Serving: 1

Nutritional Value (Approximate):

- Calories: 120
- Carbohydrates: 15g, Protein: 4g
- Healthy Fats: 6g, Fiber: 5g

Cheese and Whole Grain Crackers

Ingredients:

1 ounce cheese (cheddar or Swiss), sliced

1 serving whole grain crackers

Preparation:

1. Arrange sliced cheese on a platter.
2. Serve with whole-grain crackers.
3. Enjoy this simple and balanced snack.

Serving: 1

Nutritional Value (Approximate):

- Calories: 180
- Carbohydrates: 15g, Protein: 8g
- Healthy Fats: 10g, Fiber: 3g

Hard-Boiled Eggs with Cherry Tomatoes

Ingredients:

2 hard-boiled eggs, sliced

1/2 cup cherry tomatoes, halved

1/2 teaspoon black pepper

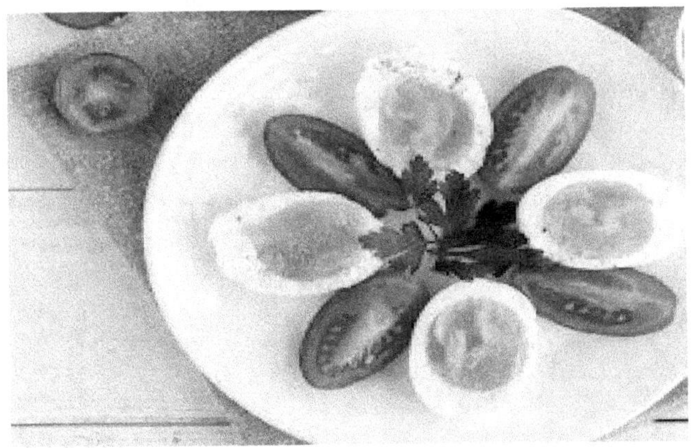

Preparation:

1. Slice hard-boiled eggs.

2. Arrange sliced eggs and cherry tomatoes on a platter.

3. Sprinkle black pepper on top.

Serving: 1

Nutritional Value (Approximate):

- Calories: 140, Carbohydrates: 5g
- Protein: 12g, Healthy Fats: 8g, Fiber: 2g

Almond Butter with Apple Slices

Ingredients:

2 tablespoons almond butter

1 medium apple, cut

Preparation:

1. Spread almond butter on apple slices.

2. Enjoy this delicious and balanced snack that mixes natural sweetness with healthy fats.

Yogurt & Granola Bowl

Ingredients:

1 cup plain Greek yogurt

1/4 cup granola (select a low-sugar alternative)

1/2 cup mixed berries (blueberries, raspberries)

1 tbsp chia seeds

Preparation:

1. In a serving bowl, layer Greek yogurt.
2. Top with granola, mixed berries, and chia seeds.
3. Mix before eating for a lovely and enjoyable snack.

Serving: 1

Nutritional Value (Approximate):

- Calories: 200

- Carbohydrates: 25g, Protein: 15g

- Healthy Fats: 6g, Fiber: 6g

Cucumber and Tuna Bites

Ingredients:

1 cucumber, cut into rounds

1 can (5 oz) tuna, drained

1 tablespoon mayonnaise (select a light or olive oil-based variant)

1 teaspoon Dijon mustard

Fresh dill for garnish (optional)

Nutritional Value (Approximate):

- Calories: 150 , Carbohydrates: 5g

- Protein: 20g, Healthy Fats: 6g, Fiber: 1g

Serving: 1 serving

Preparation:

1. In a bowl, mix drained tuna, mayonnaise, and Dijon mustard.

2. Place a dollop of the tuna mixture on each cucumber round.

3. Garnish with fresh dill if desired before serving.

These cucumber and tuna bites offer a pleasant and protein-packed snack alternative.

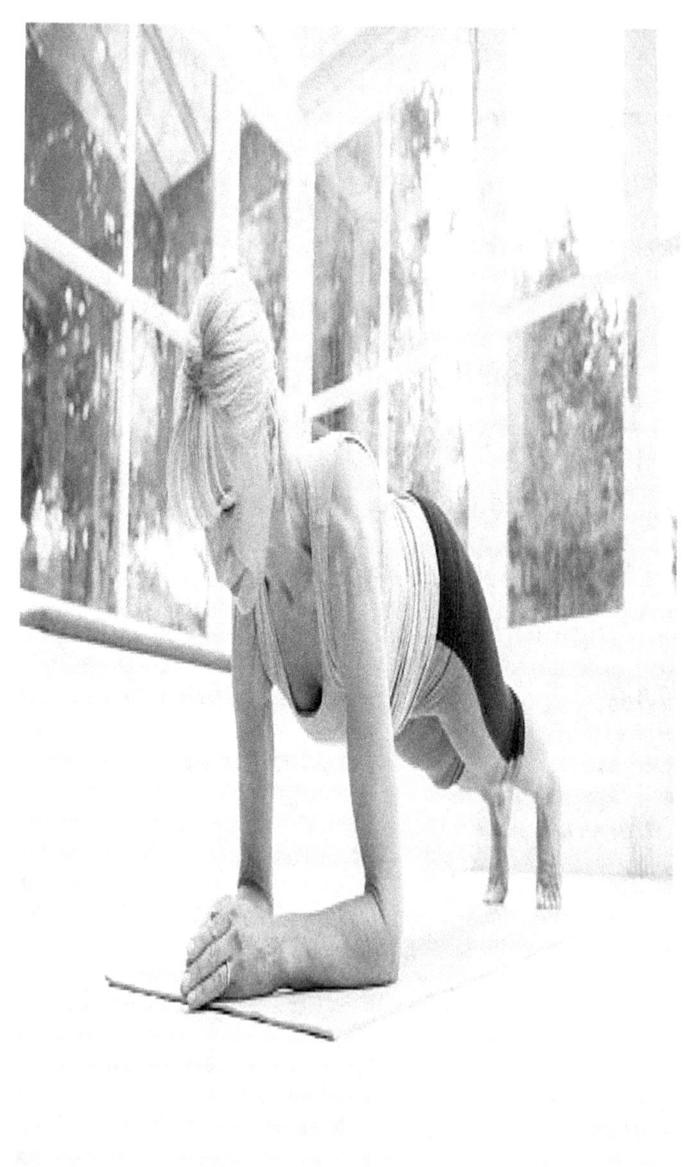

Chapter 8: Exercise Plan for Type 1 Diabetes

7-Day Exercise Plan:

Day 1:

- **Walking Exercise:**

Brisk walking for 20 minutes.

Start with a gentle warm-up, then walk at a

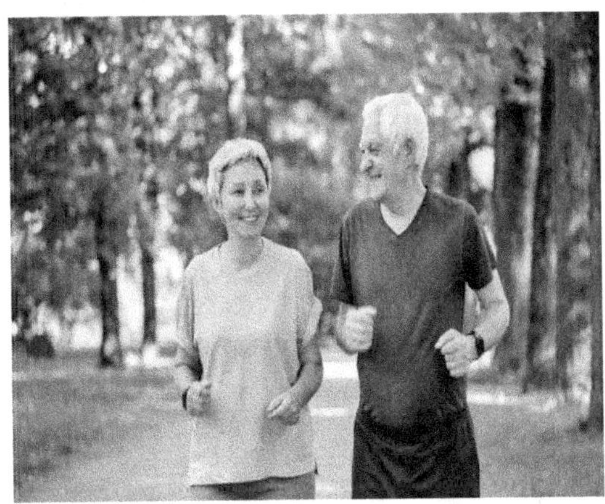

pace that gets you slightly breathless but still able to carry a conversation. Swing your arms and keep proper posture. Focus on your breathing and appreciate the fresh air.

Health Benefits:

- Cardiovascular Health: Walking improves blood circulation, decreases blood pressure, and reduces the risk of heart disease.
- Blood Sugar Control: Regular walking helps regulate blood sugar levels by boosting insulin sensitivity.
- Weight Management: It burns calories and aids in weight maintenance.
- Mental Well-being: Walking outdoors increases mood and reduces stress.

Day 2:

- ***Chair Exercises***

Seated leg raise.

Sit in a sturdy chair with your feet flat on the floor. Lift one leg straight out in front of you, hold for a few seconds, and then lower it. Repeat with the opposite leg. This helps

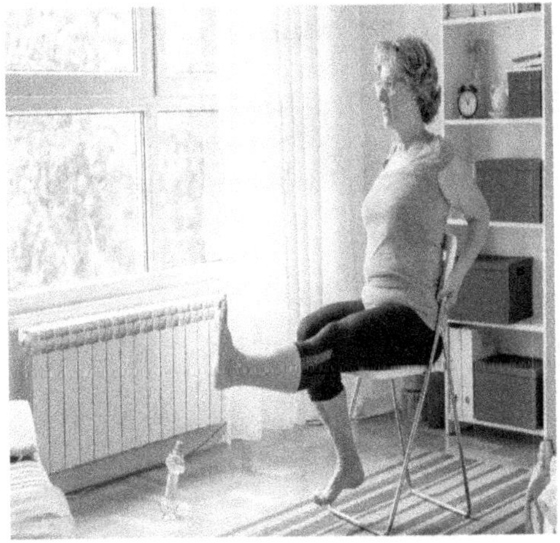

strengthen your leg muscles and promote circulation.

Health Benefits:

- Muscle Strength: Leg lifts develop leg muscles, improving mobility and balance.

- Joint Flexibility: These workouts increase joint health and flexibility.

- Blood Flow: Leg motions promote circulation, boosting general health.

- ***Resistance Band Workout Exercise: Seated rowing with a resistance band.***

Attach the resistance band to a doorknob or other stable anchor. Sit tall on your chair,

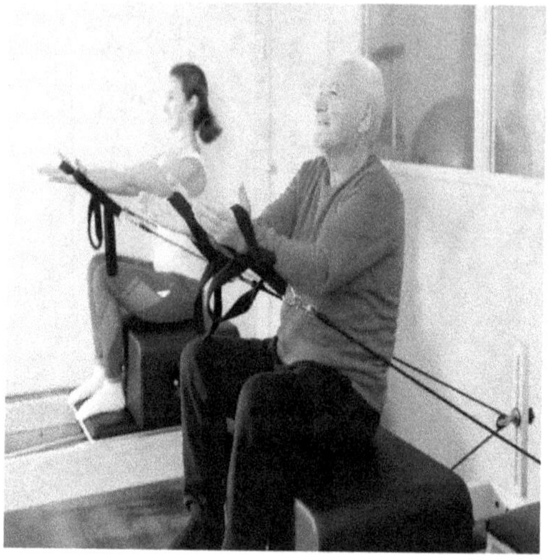

grab the band handles, and draw them toward your chest as if rowing.

This works your upper back and arms.

Health Benefits:

- Upper Body Strength: Rowing engages back, shoulder, and arm muscles.

- Posture Improvement: It helps counteract the consequences of sitting for long durations.

- Bone Health: Resistance exercises enhance bone density.

-

Balancing Practice Exercise:
Single-leg balancing.

Stand behind a strong chair or use a wall for support. Lift one foot off the ground and balance on the other leg. Hold for 10–15 seconds, then swap legs. This helps enhance balance and stability.

Health Benefits:

- Balance Enhancement: Practicing single-leg balance minimizes the danger of falls.

- Core Activation: It activates core muscles, providing stability.

- Joint Stability: Balancing on one leg strengthens ankles and knees.

Day 5:

- ***Yoga Exercise:***

Seated forward fold.

Sit on the edge of a chair with your feet flat

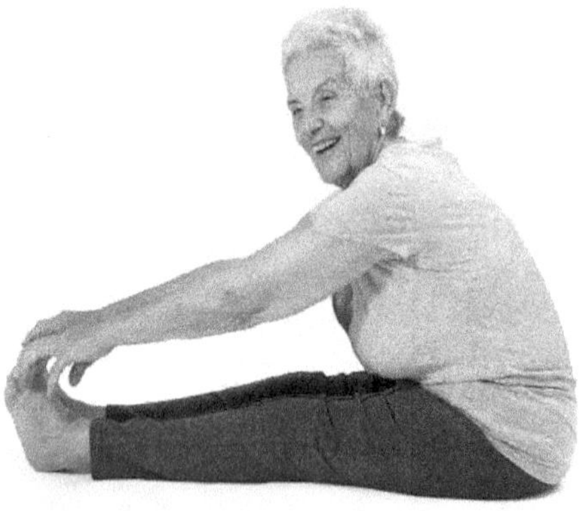

on the floor. Inhale, stretch your spine and exhale as you bend forward from your hips. Reach your hands toward your feet. Hold for a few breaths, then gently come back up. This stretches your hamstrings and lower back.

Health Benefits:

- Flexibility: Stretching hamstrings and lower back promotes general flexibility.
- Stress Reduction: Yoga improves relaxation and mental well-being.
- Digestive Health: Forward folds improve digestion.

Day 6:

- ***Stationary Bike Exercise:***

Cycling on a stationary bike.

Adjust the seat height so your knees have a slight bend when cycling. Start with a low resistance and progressively raise it. Pedal for 15–20 minutes. This is great for cardiovascular health.

Health Benefits:

- Calorie Burn: It improves weight management and supports blood sugar regulation.

<u>*Day 7:*</u>

- ***Tai Chi Exercise:***

Tai Chi movements. Tai Chi incorporates slow, flowing movements

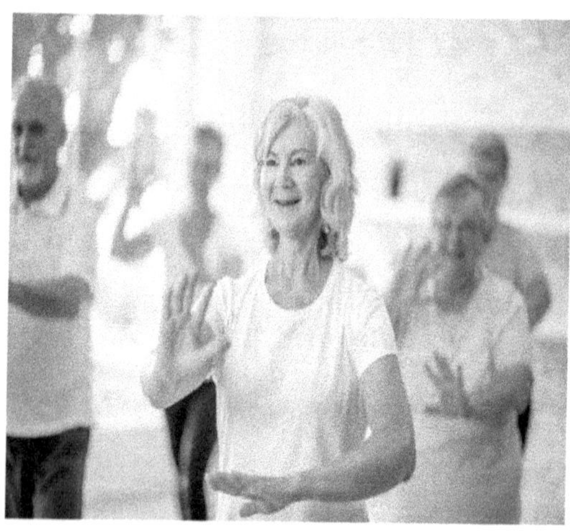

that promote balance, flexibility, and overall well-being.

Health Benefits:

Balance and Coordination: Tai Chi improves balance and minimizes the chance of falls.

Stress Reduction: Slow, flowing movements relax the mind.

Energy Flow: Tai Chi enhances the flow of vital energy (qi) in the body.

Foods and Things To Avoid:

→ Highly processed foods: Fast food, sugary snacks, and processed meals can lead to rapid spikes in blood sugar. Opt for whole, unprocessed foods.

→ Sugary Drinks and Meals: Regular sodas, fruit juices, and other sweetened beverages have the potential to produce large variations in blood sugar levels. Make your selection from sugar-free beverages, herbal tea, or water.

→ Refined Carbohydrates:White bread, white rice, and other refined carbohydrates can cause quick increases in blood sugar.

→ High-Sugar Desserts: Cakes, cookies, pastries, and candies are high in sugar and can lead to blood sugar spikes. Consider healthier dessert alternatives, like fresh fruits or sugar-free options.

Fried and Fatty Foods: Fried foods and those high in saturated fats can impact heart health. Go for healthier cooking methods like baking, grilling, or steaming.

Alcohol in Excess: Alcohol has a way of affecting blood sugar levels and interacts with diabetes medications. Consume alcohol in moderation and always with food to avoid hypoglycemia.

Things to Consider:

- ❖ Carbohydrate Monitoring: Keep track of carbohydrate intake as it directly influences blood sugar levels. Learn to count carbs in meals and snacks.

❖ Consistent Meal Timing: Establish a regular eating schedule to help manage blood sugar. Consistency in meal timing can make it easier to control glucose levels.

❖ Protein Intake: Include lean proteins in meals to help stabilize blood sugar levels.

Mediterranean vegetable skewers

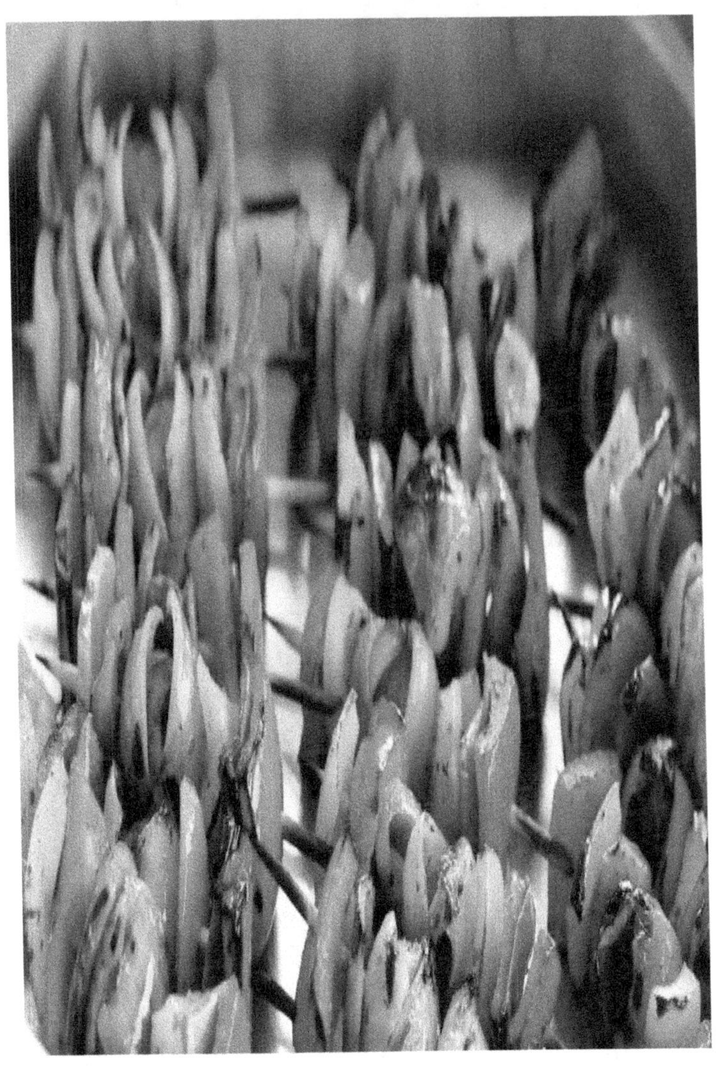

"Type 1 Diabetes Cookbook for Seniors" is not simply a collection of recipes, it is a comprehensive handbook aimed to empower and enhance the lives of seniors living with Type 1 Diabetes.

Our trip has brought us through professionally prepared meal programs, rich with nutrient needs tailored for seniors. From breakfast to dinner, each recipe not only stresses health but also highlights the pleasure of eating. We've studied diabetes kitchen basics, ingredients, and practical meal-planning tactics, ensuring that every dish is not just balanced but also delicious.

As we embrace the power of food as medicine, this cookbook stands as a companion on the road toward optimal health for seniors with Type 1 Diabetes. It is a tribute to the fact that one may relish the delight of eating while properly controlling diabetes through conscious, nutritional choices. With a focus on simplicity, variety, and the use of diabetes-friendly ingredients, this cookbook intends to encourage a lifetime commitment to well-being.

Remember, the path to healthy living is a personal journey, and this cookbook is a guide to making that trip delectable, fun, and sustainable. May each recipe assist not only in better diabetes management but also in a fulfilling and vibrant existence for every senior embracing the culinary delights within these pages? Cheers to excellent health and the pleasure of nourishing both body and soul!